Masculinity and Sexuality

Selected Topics in the Psychology of Men

Review of Psychiatry Series
John M. Oldham, M.D., and
Michelle B. Riba, M.D.
Series Editors

Masculinity and Sexuality

Selected Topics in the Psychology of Men

EDITED BY

**Richard C. Friedman, M.D., and
Jennifer I. Downey, M.D.**

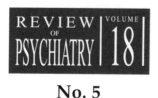

REVIEW OF PSYCHIATRY | VOLUME 18

No. 5

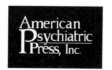

American Psychiatric Press, Inc.

Washington, DC
London, England

Copyright © 1999 American Psychiatric Press, Inc.

02 01 00 99   4 3 2 1

ALL RIGHTS RESERVED

Manufactured in the United States of America on acid-free paper

American Psychiatric Press, Inc.
1400 K Street, N.W.
Washington, DC 20005
www.appi.org

The correct citation for this book is

> Friedman RC, Downey JI (eds.): *Masculinity and Sexuality: Selected Topics in the Psychology of Men* (Review of Psychiatry Series; Oldham JO and Riba MB, series eds.). Washington, DC, American Psychiatric Press, 1999

Library of Congress Cataloging-in-Publication Data
Masculinity and sexuality : selected topics in the psychology of men /
    edited by Richard C. Friedman and Jennifer I. Downey.
        p.   cm. — (Review of psychiatry series ; v. 18, no. 5)
    Includes bibliographical references and index.
    ISBN 0-88048-962-6
    1. Men—Mental health.   2. Men—Sexual behavior.   3. Men—
Psychology.   I. Friedman, Richard C., 1941–   .   II. Downey,
Jennifer I.   III. Series.
    [DNLM: 1. Men—psychology.   2. Sex behavior.   HQ 28 M395 1999]
RC451.4.M45M37   1999
616.89' 0082—dc21
DNLM/DLC
for Library of Congress   99-26611
                                                                                    CIP

British Library Cataloguing in Publication Data
A CIP record is available from the British Library.

Contents

Contributors   *ix*

Introduction to the Review of
Psychiatry Series   *xi*
    John M. Oldham, M.D., and
    Michelle B. Riba, M.D., Series Editors

Foreword   *xiii*
    Richard C. Friedman, M.D., and
    Jennifer I. Downey, M.D.

Chapter 1
Sexual Fantasy and Behavior:
Selected Clinical Issues   **1**
    Richard C. Friedman, M.D., and
    Jennifer I. Downey, M.D.
Sexual Fantasy   2
Sexuality in the Psychotherapeutic Situation   6
Relationship Between Sexual Fantasy and
    Sexual Activity   13
Sexual Impulsivity and Compulsivity   14
Special Clinical Problems in Men With
    Severe Personality Disorders   21
Sexual Orientation Conversion   23
Conclusion   24
References   25

Chapter 2
Male Heterosexuality   **29**
    Stephen B. Levine, M.D.
The Evolution of Heterosexuality   30
Default Heterosexuality   32
The Concept of Male Heterosexual
    Developmental Failure   36

Common Manifestations of Heterosexual
    Developmental Failures   42
Intimacy Skills   47
References   52

Chapter 3

**Evaluation and Treatment of
Erectile Dysfunction**   **55**

*Stanley E. Althof, Ph.D., and
Allen D. Seftel, M.D.*

Nosology: Impotence Versus Erectile
    Dysfunction   56
Prevalence and Medical Risk Factors   57
Physiology of Erection   58
Integration of Biological and Psychiatric Theories:
    The Interactive Etiologic Model Paradigm   65
Process of Care Model   66
New Roles for Mental Health Clinicians   78
The Future   81
References   81

Chapter 4

**Fatherhood as a Transformation
of the Self: Steps Toward a New
Psychology of Men**   **89**

William S. Pollack, Ph.D.

Rethinking Development: Men and Women   92
Early Development   92
Beyond Freud—Beneath the
    Oedipus Complex   93
A Normative (Gender-Linked)
    Developmental Trauma   94
The Balancing Act: The "I" and the "We"   96
Fatherhood: A Second Chance   99
Good-Enough Fathering:
    Fathering as a Developmental Phase   101
Personal Transformations   104
Inhibitions and Interruptions in the
    Transition to Fatherhood   107

What Do Men (and Boys) Really Need?   109
Conclusion   111
References   113

Chapter 5
**Casualties of Recovered Memory Therapy:
The Impact of False Allegations of
Incest on Accused Fathers   115**
 Harold I. Lief, M.D., and
 Janet M. Fetkewicz, M.A.
Overview   117
Repression   117
Recovery of Memories   118
False Memory Syndrome   120
Theoretical Issues   122
Role of Suggestion   123
Mutually Reinforcing Beliefs   124
Therapeutic Assumptions   126
Impact of an Accusation   128
Interviews With Accused Fathers   131
Discussion   136
Conclusion   138
References   138

Afterword   *143*
 Richard C. Friedman, M.D., and
 Jennifer I. Downey, M.D.

Index   *145*

Contributors

Stanley E. Althof, Ph.D.   Associate Professor of Psychology, Case Western Reserve University School of Medicine; Staff Psychologist, University Hospitals of Cleveland; and Co-director, Center for Marital and Sexual Health, Cleveland, Ohio

Jennifer I. Downey, M.D.   Associate Clinical Professor of Psychiatry and Director, Psycho-oncology, Herbert Irving Comprehensive Cancer Center, Columbia University College of Physicians and Surgeons, New York, New York

Janet M. Fetkewicz, M.A.   Research Assistant, False Memory Syndrome Foundation, Philadelphia, Pennsylvania

Richard C. Friedman, M.D.   Clinical Professor of Psychiatry, Cornell University School of Medicine; and Lecturer, Columbia University College of Physicians and Surgeons, New York, New York

Stephen B. Levine, M.D.   Clinical Professor, Case Western Reserve University School of Medicine, Cleveland, Ohio; and Co-Director, Center for Marital and Sexual Health, Beachwood, Ohio

Harold I. Lief, M.D.   Emeritus Professor of Psychiatry, University of Pennsylvania; and Clinical Professor of Psychiatry, Thomas Jefferson Medical College, Philadelphia, Pennsylvania

John M. Oldham, M.D.   Director, New York State Psychiatric Institute; and Dollard Professor and Vice Chairman, Department of Psychiatry, Columbia University College of Physicians and Surgeons, New York, New York

William S. Pollack, Ph.D.   Director, Center for Men, McLean Hospital; and Assistant Clinical Professor, Department of Psychiatry, Harvard Medical School, Belmont, Massachusetts

Michelle B. Riba, M.D.   Clinical Associate Professor of Psychiatry and Associate Chair for Education and Academic Affairs, Department of Psychiatry, University of Michigan Health System, Ann Arbor, Michigan

Allen D. Seftel, M.D.   Associate Professor of Urology, Case Western Reserve University School of Medicine; and Attending Urologist, University Hospitals of Cleveland and the Cleveland Veterans Administration Medical Center, Cleveland, Ohio

Introduction to the Review of Psychiatry Series

John M. Oldham, M.D., and
Michelle B. Riba, M.D., Series Editors

As this century and millennium come to a close, it seems a universal impulse to pause and "take stock." Any time is a good time to do this, of course, but the big round number 2000 just over the horizon seems a special one. It turns out to be, in our opinion, quite a good time for the field of psychiatry. Although a great deal more work lies ahead, we have made substantial progress in the fight for parity, with stronger partnerships having been built among clinicians, patients, families, and advocates. We are hopefully past the most extreme swing of the pendulum of managed care overcontrol, with a new, quite strong professional voice emerging to articulate and define evidence-based practice guidelines and best practices and to set performance standards and develop quality and outcome indicators for good clinical care.

The explosion of knowledge in neuroscience, meanwhile, only accelerates, with its accompanying breathtaking advances in technology. As more is learned about the circuitry of the brain, we obtain a clearer understanding of neurodevelopment gone awry in vulnerable populations such as those at risk to develop schizophrenia. But as we learn more about the brain's "hard-wiring," an entire frontier of information is unfolding, demonstrating an unprecedented plasticity of the brain. In turn, the sensitive, bidirectional interplay between biology and the environment becomes the name of the game.

In the context of these and many other features of our present landscape, we have chosen for this year's Annual Review a sampling of the latest knowledge and thinking from clinical practice and from the laboratory: 1) countertransference issues in psychiatric treatment, 2) disruptive behavior disorders in children and adolescents, 3) gender differences in mood and anxiety disorders,

4) molecular biology of schizophrenia, and 5) masculinity and sexuality.

We are grateful to our section editors and our authors, who worked hard and successfully to produce the text material. As well, we are indebted to Carol Nadelson, M.D.; Claire Reinburg; Pamela Harley; Ron McMillen; and the entire American Psychiatric Press, Inc., staff. And the entire project would not have been possible without the steady help of Sam McGowan and Linda Gacioch.

Foreword

Richard C. Friedman, M.D., and
Jennifer I. Downey, M.D.

The five chapters in this volume dealing with masculinity and male sexuality remind us that the practice of psychiatry is a human enterprise, a fact sometimes overlooked because of recent economic pressures on health care delivery. Sexual experiences and attitudes of patients and therapists influence symptoms, treatment, and outcome across diverse diagnostic categories.

All men experience sexual thoughts, impulses, and desires. In the first chapter, Friedman and Downey discuss the way that these thoughts, impulses, and desires are organized into erotic fantasies, or personal narratives suffused with sexual emotion. They review the fundamental differences that exist between the way men and women experience sexual fantasy. Long before the discipline of psychiatry existed, philosophers and artists recognized that the urge to gratify erotic desire frequently conflicted with the sense of social responsibility. The authors discuss the clinical manifestations of conflict between impulse and conscience and illustrate these manifestations with vignettes that put an emphasis on impulsive/compulsive and self-destructive sexual activity. A particularly important point of this chapter is that a sexual history should be a routine part of the assessment of every patient.

In the second chapter, Levine discusses heterosexuality, an area somewhat neglected in contemporary psychiatry. In Levine's words:

> Modern psychiatry, in its romance with the brain's anatomic and biochemical dimensions, has moved away from the idea that psychiatric diagnoses have anything to do with psychological development and love.

Levine suggests that heterosexuality is best conceptualized as part of a developmental line that includes the capacity for intimacy and love. He points out that absent the latter, men "default" to a state in which they seek sexual activity with women but not with a particular woman who is appreciated as an individual. Levine considers this a developmental failure and argues that many psychiatric symptoms and disorders can result from it. Whether or not one agrees with his paradigm, it is difficult to discount the importance of assessing the patient's capacity for intimacy and love as part of an adequate psychiatric evaluation, in addition to the specific symptoms that together characterize DSM-IV Axis I and Axis II disorders. Although Levine's chapter focuses on heterosexuality, assessment of the capacity for intimacy and love is certainly also indicated for patients whose sexual orientation is bisexual or homosexual.

In the history of medicine, a few drugs stand above others in their therapeutic impact and social consequences. Aspirin and penicillin are in this category, and more recently, sildenafil citrate (Viagra) has attracted enormous attention. In their chapter on erectile dysfunction, Althof and Seftel review the physiology of male sexual function and explain the pharmacology of sildenafil as part of a more inclusive discussion of pharmacotherapy of sexual dysfunction. They then outline a paradigm for integrating the biological and psychological factors that together influence male sexual dysfunction. Never losing sight of the necessity to understand and offer treatment to individuals and couples, the authors outline new roles for mental health clinicians in light of recent advances of knowledge about human sexuality.

One of the most important and transforming influences on men's development is fatherhood; however, only recently has psychoanalytic psychology begun to attend seriously to the many meanings and effects of fatherhood. In his chapter, Pollack discusses fatherhood from the perspective of psychoanalytic self psychology and in the context of recent advances in gender psychology. The sexes differ in the way each experiences and expresses affiliative behavior toward children. Men are more likely to experience shared activities as intimate, whereas women are more likely to be directly physically demonstrative. Pollack emphasizes that the experience of fatherhood is often as important as, or more important than, career achievement in self-assessment of masculine adequacy. He notes that the capacity of men to be nurturant and fatherly extends beyond their children and is certainly present in many men who are not fathers. His discussion of the role of fatherhood in psychological development during adulthood directs attention to an area worthy of scrutiny and research in the future.

In their chapter on casualties of recovered memory therapy, Lief and Fetkewicz discuss the victimization of fathers by children who make false allegations of sexual abuse. The authors point out that actual sexual abuse is a serious problem and that its psychiatric consequences have been documented extensively. The situation they discuss, however, is quite different. In recent years some psychotherapists have subtly influenced patients to "recall memories" allegedly repressed—which presumably account for the patients' psychiatric symptoms and which involve childhood sexual molestation by a parent. Lief and Fetkewicz observe that these alleged memories are often false beliefs—the so-called traumatic sexual events never occurred. The authors review the phenomenon in which the accusation of childhood sexual abuse is repudiated by the accuser. They attribute the wave of accusations associated with (alleged) "recovered memories," which peaked in the 1980s, to increased awareness of childhood sexual abuse by organizations, institutions, and governmental agencies; a widespread tendency in American society at that time to idealize "victims"; the burgeoning of diverse types of self-help groups; and the sociopolitical power of radical feminism. Their sobering chapter raises serious questions about the abuse of men by women.

Chapter 1

Sexual Fantasy and Behavior: Selected Clinical Issues

Richard C. Friedman, M.D., and
Jennifer I. Downey, M.D.

A person's sexual life consists of mental experience and sexual activity with others. Much nonsexual experience is composed of fantasy, and this also is true of sexual experience. In order to understand sexual fantasy—a core component of sexual experience—it is necessary to first consider more general aspects of fantasy.

Fantasies are stories that we tell ourselves for a variety of reasons. They soothe us when our nerves are jangled, help stabilize our self-esteem, allow us to imagine future courses of action, and fulfill wishes (consider the fictional character Walter Mitty, who becomes a fighter pilot through his fantasies). A key function of fantasy during childhood, for example, is to provide a script for role rehearsal. Children play house, or doctor, or cops and robbers, imagining themselves in adult roles that they endow with the luster of romantic idealization (Person 1995). Freud pointed out that people seem to have an innate tendency to keep their fantasies private, even secret, as if they were ashamed of the childish or socially unacceptable aspects of self-revelation that occur in these fantasies.

> The adult . . . is ashamed of his phantasies and hides them from other people. He cherishes his phantasies as his most intimate possessions, and as a rule he would rather confess his misdeeds than tell anyone his phantasies. It may come about that for that reason he believes he is the only person who invents such phantasies and has no idea that creations of this kind are widespread among other people. (Freud 1907/1989, p. 438)

The sense of shame that Freud observed about fantasies in general is often especially true of sexual fantasies. From the perspective of information processing, fantasies allow us to represent large amounts of information in a textured narrative structure. Mental processes, unlike computer programs, for example, are not organized in a linear, logical manner. The unique blend of thoughts, feelings, memories, perceptions, symbolic representational thinking, and sense of drama that characterizes fantasy is so complex that no computer appears capable of it, at least at present. This is illustrated dramatically by the well-publicized contest between the computer called Deep Blue and the world chess champion Kasparov. Deep Blue defeated Kasparov because of its almost limitless capacity to consider alternative moves that might occur in the future. In that sense, some observers might say that Deep Blue "fantasized" about future possibilities of action. Deep Blue did not, however, chuckle in delicious anticipation of a clever move or say to itself (as far as we know), "Now I've got you, you sonofabitch." Similarly, it did not experience shame and anxiety that it might not live up to the expectations of earlier generations of computers, nor for that matter did it become distracted by sexual fantasies.

Sexual Fantasy

Among forms of fantasy in men, sexual fantasy is unique because it depends on the occurrence of explicitly sexual feelings. Sexual lust is a specific emotion like fear, joy, anger, or sadness. The capacity of adults to experience the sense of sexual emotion, a necessary component of what is usually termed sexual desire, arousal, or excitement, depends on the presence of adequate blood levels of androgen. Sexual fantasies are virtually eliminated by certain antiandrogenic pharmacologic agents, such as cyproterone acetate (Rosen and Beck 1988). Lustful sexual feeling depends on biochemical and physiologic processes that occur throughout the body, especially in the brain (Paredes and Baum 1997; Rosen and Leiblum 1992). The same psychophysiologic changes occur in all men during the sexual response cycle (Masters and Johnson 1966). However, identical sexual fantasies do not occur in all men.

Men in particular subgroups experience specific types of sexual fantasies that are different from those experienced by men in other subgroups. In thinking about this concept, consider the analogy of the theater. The entire set of sexual fantasies in the human repertoire of mental experience may be likened to all plays performed in New York City. Large audiences attend each play, but each play is different. The analogy goes only so far, however, because an average theatergoer has the capacity to be involved in the other plays, should he happen to attend them. This is not the case with sexual fantasy. The scenarios that constitute sexual fantasies appear to have unique abilities to arouse specific groups of men. Exposure to other types of fantasies (i.e., the play next door, according to our analogy) tends to be responded to with indifference. A particular man tends to play out in his mind the same type of sexual fantasy over and over again for his entire sexual life. For example, a heterosexual man might imagine the image of a nude woman, a woman undressing or being undressed, and so on, whereas a gay man might imagine the image of a nude man. Exposure of the heterosexual to a nude man and the homosexual to a nude woman will not stimulate sexual interest or arousal, and sexual emotion will not be experienced (Freund et al. 1974).

Person (1988) has used the term "sexprint" to describe this phenomenon, whereas Money (1988) has used the expression "lovemap." No matter what terminology is used, the central concept that these investigators (and others) agree about is that in men sexual fantasy appears to act as a limit on possible imagined constructs. The limit describes a universe that may be quite large, or so narrow and rigidly bounded that the patient meets criteria for a paraphilia. (The paraphilias constitute a discrete set of disorders whose diagnosis and treatment we do not discuss in this chapter. We refer interested readers to Abel et al. [1992] and Bradford and Greenberg [1996].)

A number of investigators have pointed out that among males the time during the life cycle when the boundaries of the subjectively experienced sexual domain (i.e., the sexprint or lovemap) are set appears to be childhood, sometime prior to puberty (Friedman 1988; Money and Ehrhardt 1972). McClintock and Herdt

(1996) have noted that the peak age at which this occurs appears to coincide with adrenarche, again indicating the importance of androgens in the subjective sexual experience.

Sex Differences in Sexual Fantasy

Sexual fantasies have the capacity to perform the same psychological functions as other types of fantasies (e.g., wish fulfillment, self-soothing). However, they also motivate sexual activity, including masturbation and interpersonal sexual activity. The determinants, characteristics, and functions of sexual fantasy differ between men and women. These differences must be considered in conceptualizing heterosexual relationships. Whereas women need not be sexually aroused nor motivated by sexual fantasy, men need to be in order to engage in interpersonal sexual activity. Another important sex difference, probably attributable to neuroendocrine differences between the sexes, is that asexual states of mind are experienced far less commonly by men than women (Laan and Everaerd 1995; Seidman and Rieder 1994). Repetitive, insistent, persistent sexual arousal with its often attendant fantasies is experienced by virtually all men at least between puberty and middle age and by many men in later life. Women are much more diverse in this regard. Although some women seem to experience sexual fantasies with the same frequency as do men, most women do not.

At all ages males participate in sexual activity with greater frequency than do females, no matter what type of activity is involved. They also have more sexual partners in the course of a lifetime (Billy et al. 1993; Blumstein and Schwartz 1983; Friedman and Downey 1994; Seidman and Rieder 1994). As a group, men tend to value monogamy less than do women and also tend to place less of a premium on intimacy or love as a precondition for sexual activity. In heterosexual relationships, men are more likely than women to value the relationship in terms of the quality of sexuality in it, whereas women are more likely than men to evaluate the sexuality in terms of the quality of the relationship. This difference is often expressed by heterosexual partners who seek couple's counseling. The man is likely to complain that the couple's sexual life is impoverished; the woman that their emotional life is the problem. Embattled with each other, the man is likely to argue that the quality of their emotional life would improve if sexual contact were more frequent and satisfying. The woman, in contrast, is likely to respond that she would feel like participating in sexual activity more frequently if the man were more emotionally available and communicative, that is, if the couple's emotional life created an atmosphere in which her sexual desire could emerge.

Masculine self-esteem tends to be integrated with a man's erotic life in an immediate and direct way. The situation is much more diverse among women. It is probably safe to conclude that as a general rule feminine self-esteem is not integrated with the erotic life of most women in quite the same immediate way, although there is much overlap between the sexes with regard to this behavioral dimension (Hatfield and Rapson 1993; Laan and Everaerd 1995; Tyson 1994).

Sexual Orientation

By *sexual orientation* we mean the gender of the sexual object that leads to sexual arousal—same sex, opposite sex, or both. Although sexual fantasies may be categorized similarly, they are not sharply bounded from each other. As Kinsey and colleagues pointed out, the boundaries of one group fade into those of the adjacent one, so that the homosexual-heterosexual balance of fantasies or activity appears to fall along a continuum (Kinsey et al. 1948). At the poles of the continuum, however, are individuals whose lifelong sexual fantasy programming has been exclusively heterosexual or homosexual. In terms of the percentage, the heterosexual group is large and the homosexual group small, consisting of 1%–2% of the male population. This is nonetheless a large number of people in terms of absolute numbers. A person's orienting sexual fantasies may or may not be congruent with his perceived sense of self-identity and social role with others (that one is homosexual, heterosexual, or bisexual). In American culture the category of *bisexual* is not commonly accepted, and people tend to group themselves into one of two categories: gay or heterosexual. Many gay people have heterosexual fantasies, and about 20% are or have been married. Many people considered heterosexual nonetheless experience homosexual fantasies (Friedman and Downey 1994). Celibate people experience the same range of sexually orienting fantasies as those who are sexually active with others.

Sexuality in the Psychotherapeutic Situation

There are many forms of psychotherapy, and in this chapter we discuss only those that are psychodynamically oriented. Psychodynamic psychotherapies may be brief or lengthy; crisis oriented or not; and directed at uncovering repressed unconscious (e.g., warded-off) memories in order to better understand the influence of the distant past on the present, or—to the contrary—focused on the "here and now." They may or may not utilize free association and interpretation of dreams, and they may or may not use as a learning tool the patient's irrationally determined attitudes toward the therapist—termed *transference* by Freud (Freud 1900/1953; Moore and Fine 1995). Formal psychoanalysis would be found at one extreme of a continuum representing some of these behavioral dimensions; time-limited brief psychotherapy would be found at the other extreme.

All psychodynamically oriented psychotherapies share a few basic assumptions:

- All experience has meanings that are both conscious and unconscious.
- At least some experience and activity are unconsciously motivated.
- Aspects of past and imagined experience deemed particularly meaningful are expressed symbolically, in disguised fashion, in the psychological experience of the present. Therefore, present experience and activity are influenced by the past, although in ways not necessarily immediately apparent to the individual (Olds 1994).
- The therapist's understanding of the relationship between conscious and unconscious processes, when applied cor-

rectly in the treatment situation, can have beneficial effects.

- Psychotherapy occurs within the context of a specific type of professional relationship with rules that govern its practical (including financial) and ethical operations. These assumptions create a common way of looking at behavior among dynamic psychotherapists who may differ on numerous other issues (Lazar 1997; Ursano et al. 1998).

People who seek psychotherapy vary with regard to the degree of their impairment of psychological functioning. More severely impaired patients may have a number of Axis I and Axis II psychiatric diagnoses (according to the *Diagnostic and Statistical Manual of Mental Disorders,* Fourth Edition [DSM-IV] [American Psychiatric Association 1994]). They may have histories of psychiatric hospitalizations or suicide attempts and early life histories of severe abuse (including sexual abuse) or neglect. These patients would have a low overall level of functioning on Axis V, indicated in DSM-IV terms by a low Global Assessment of Functioning (GAF) score. Toward the other end of the spectrum of severity are those patients who experience painful symptoms but who do not meet criteria for a specific psychiatric diagnosis. These patients tend to have a higher GAF score than those in the former group. People across the entire spectrum seek relief from psychic pain and improvement in their capacity to love, work, and experience pleasure (including sexual pleasure) and joy. In recent years dramatic progress in psychopharmacology has led to an increase in the application of combined psychotherapeutic and psychopharmacologic treatments. We assume that the patients in psychotherapy who are discussed in this chapter may or may not be receiving concurrent psychopharmacologic treatment (Friedman et al. 1998; Lazar 1997).

Initial Assessment

A sexual history should be an integral component of the assessment of all psychotherapy patients. In the initial interview therapist and patient are strangers to one another, and it is understandable that the patient might be guarded about discussing, with someone he or she does not know, aspects of his or her inner life that may be a source of shame. Even so, some data about the patient's sexual motivations and activities can usually be elicited. This information is helpful in conceptualizing the patient's general adaptational level. For example, it is generally possible to determine whether a patient has been interpersonally sexually active recently and to assess—at least in a preliminary fashion—orienting sexual fantasies. People have diverse responses to simple, open-ended questions such as, "Can you tell me something about your sexual life?" Although less experienced clinicians sometimes fear that even mentioning sex is likely to be seen as intrusive or invasive, this is rarely the case. In fact, most people welcome the opportunity to discuss their sexuality and have little opportunity to do so in day-to-day life. Many patients come to the therapeutic situation seeking information or reassurance about questions related to sex, even though they do not identify such concerns in their chief complaint.

Questions that the authors have been asked in the initial interview include the following: "Can someone masturbate too much and damage themselves?" "My 45-year-old husband wants sex every day. Don't you think he is oversexed?" "Is anal intercourse normal?" "Is HIV transmissible by kissing?" "Can people have sexual intercourse during pregnancy?" and "I have had two heart attacks. Will sex give me another?" Thus in the very first interview patients may be eager to discuss with the therapist a wide-ranging set of issues pertaining to sexuality. Many other aspects of the patient's sexual history may emerge once a therapeutic working alliance has developed. In general, the more the patient is ashamed of sexual memories and fantasies, the more time will be necessary before they can be verbalized.

It is often difficult to obtain historical material about sexuality in the present socioeconomic climate within which psychotherapy is practiced because external financial constraints press for rapid treatment oriented around immediate symptom relief. It may even be difficult for some therapists to understand why a sexual history is relevant in the assessment of a patient who comes for help with an apparently unrelated chief complaint such as an eating disorder or a depression that the patient attributes to vocational failure. People do not experience symptoms in a compartmentalized way, however, and their sexual lives contribute to and are affected by their difficulties, no matter what form these difficulties might take. Some symptoms may be initially experienced in such a way as to avoid the sexually conflictual memories and fantasies that contribute to their etiology.

Therapists today sometimes have difficulties that eerily reproduce those faced by Freud more than 100 years ago. His patients had paralyzed limbs, and their chief complaint was neurologic, not psychological. It seemed unreasonable to the physicians of Freud's time that neurologic complaints could be caused by psychological conflicts. Freud demonstrated to the contrary that the difficulties were not only psychological but sexual in nature, thus giving birth to psychoanalysis. He initially thought that his so-called hysterical patients had all been sexually abused by their fathers but soon gave up this idea and instead suggested that their psychological suffering was attributable to sexual fantasies, that is, to unacceptable wishes (Freud 1896/1962, 1900/1953; Moore and Fine 1995; Person 1995).

Many modern therapists, strongly encouraged to limit their attentions to the patient's identified complaint, are in a situation similar to that of the 19th-century neurologists who vainly sought a neurologic cause for what appeared to be a neurologic problem. With regard to modern patients, histories of childhood sexual abuse, incestuous activity between siblings, extramarital sexual activity, paraphiliac fantasies and activities, and other sexual activities that the patient finds incompatible with his conscience structure might take weeks or months to emerge and might contribute in a disguised way to the symptoms of Axis I and Axis II psychiatric disorders (Friedman 1998).

Countertransference Difficulties That Inhibit Male Patients From Disclosing Their Sexual Fantasies

In a narrow sense, the term *countertransference* connotes the tendency of therapists to respond to patients in inappropriate, unconscious ways because of unresolved conflicts about the therapist's family of origin. In general usage, however, a somewhat broader meaning is usually adopted. In this sense, countertransference signifies a stance toward the patient that is unconsciously motivated to satisfy the therapist's needs rather than the requirements of the therapeutic situation (Moore and Fine 1995; Ursano et al. 1998). A common manifestation of countertransference difficulties occurs when therapists express negative attitudes about the sexual fantasies or activities of their patients. The therapists are unaware that they are expressing moral indignation and disapproval via responses that they consider therapeutically appropriate. Some therapists with this type of difficulty have values that are more or less conventional. Marriage and childrearing are positively sanctioned, and the traditional emblems of middle class life are highly valued. There may be a subtle tendency for therapists to idealize aspects of their own lifestyle and to equate these with psychological health. Consider, for example, the following vignette:

> Mr. A was a 24-year-old graduate student who consulted a male psychotherapist for anxiety relating to his recent relocation from a small southern town to an urban center in the Northeast. Throughout his life, Mr. A had experienced sexual fantasies and attractions only toward other boys and men, although his homosexual experience was limited to a few episodes of mutual masturbation because he had always feared exposure in the college town from which he came. Exhilarated by the freedom of living in a community that afforded more privacy, Mr. A began to spend Friday nights going to clubs where he would occasionally engage in sexual activity with men he had just met. He and his partners always used condoms, and he viewed this behavior as something he wanted to try but intended to stop when he found a man with whom he could share his life. Still, the psychiatrist objected, saying that sex was not like shaking hands or brushing teeth. Rather it should be enjoyed in the context of an intimate, loving relationship. Feeling morally censured, Mr. A's anxiety symptoms increased.

The preceding vignette illustrates the complex moral field in which clinicians practice psychotherapy. Mr. A's sexual behavior may indeed be a symptom of pathologic narcissism and a persistent inability to form meaningful relationships. Alternatively, it might be part of Mr. A's feeling of exuberance in response to being free at last to act on his homosexual identity and desires. A variety of other meanings might also be appropriate depending on details of the individual case. In this situation, the therapist imposed his personal standard of morality that only relational or procreational sex is healthy and that recreational sexuality is to be condemned.

Many therapists have intense convictions that interpersonal sexual activity should ideally occur between loving partners. Others might morally condemn extramarital affairs, activities with prostitutes, use of pornography, group sex activity—in short, sexual activities and values that are far from their own. When therapists relinquish an accepting, nonjudgmental stance, the clinical situation becomes contaminated in a psychological sense analogous to the contamination of a sterile environment by an improperly prepared surgeon. Patients may decide not to discuss their sexual fantasies in treatment because they fear disapproval. Such patients may experience intractable nonsexual symptoms (e.g., chronic severe depression, recurrent eating disorders, episodic self-mutilation, substance abuse, severe anxiety) for reasons of which the therapist is unaware. In these therapeutic situations there is a tendency for a pathologic version of splitting—a defense utilized by patients with borderline personality disorder (Kernberg 1976, 1984, 1995)—to be reinforced inadvertently. Thus the patient experiences the idealized therapist as "all good" and the self as "all bad," devalued because of recurrent unacceptable sexual fantasies.

Other patients may adopt their therapists' values in a compliant but superficial way. They then carry out self-destructive acts motivated by these values, although the self-destructive intent of these acts is perceived neither by the patient nor by the therapist. A common example involves gay patients who are themselves homophobic and whose therapists inappropriately idealize the institution of heterosexual marriage. Such patients may enter marriages that end badly for themselves and their spouses (Isay 1989, 1996). Inappropriate idealization of the institution of marriage also occurs with heterosexual patients and may lead to similarly unfortunate consequences.

Conventional therapists and unconventional patients are by no means the only commonly occurring pattern. Precisely the opposite occurs frequently—the patient may be highly conventional and experience an internal need to have a marital partner, children, and the material possessions, status, and emblems of conventional life. The therapist, much less conventional, cannot empathize with the patient's idealization of traditional values.

Moral censure is not the only countertransference problem that leads patients to inhibit verbalization of their sexual fantasies. Another major type of difficulty occurs when the patient's sexual fantasies arouse intense anxiety in the therapist. By itself, this is not necessarily a sign of countertransference difficulty. It only becomes so when the therapist's conduct becomes in some way inappropriate, motivated by personal needs to diminish anxiety in the therapeutic situation. The reasons for countertransference anxiety depend on the characteristics of both the patient's and the therapist's sexual fantasies and activities (including sexual orientation); the degree to which the therapist feels threatened by the patient's and his or her own sexual fantasies; and the degree to which the therapist feels satisfied or frustrated regarding his or her sexual life. Consider the following vignette:

> Mr. B was an attractive, successful 40-year-old novelist who consulted a female psychiatrist for a grief reaction complicated by depression following the death of his wife in an automobile accident. As Mr. B's depressive symptoms remitted on a regimen of medication and supportive psychotherapy, he began to use the sessions to discuss his loneliness and desire to meet women. Mr. B expressed the belief that he had to "make up for lost time" because he had married quite young and had had little sexual experience except with his wife. He began to discuss his preoccupation with how to seduce women and to review in some detail the mechanical aspects of the sexual relationships in which he found himself. He wondered how to decide when to enter his partner, how long he should keep an erection before orgasm, and how he could tell when his partner was satisfied. He said to the therapist, "You're a woman. Can't you tell me these things?" Mr. B's psychi-

atrist found herself feeling extremely ill at ease with these demands and wondered whether "how to seduce women" was an appropriate topic for the sessions. Anxious about her patient's sexuality, she became unaccustomedly indecisive about the nature of a proper therapeutic intervention.

Another important cause of therapist anxiety is when the therapist is the object of the patient's sexual fantasies. This often occurs when the therapist's gender is in keeping with the patient's sexual orientation (e.g., when the therapist is a woman and the patient is a heterosexual man); however, this is not always the case. Gay male patients with little or no heterosexual interest may develop erotic fantasies directed at their female therapists, and heterosexual men with little or no homosexual interest may experience the same toward male therapists. Although these responses occur often enough, they tend to be unpredictable, and often no sexual interest is expressed toward the therapist. Carrying out productive therapeutic work in the setting of an intensely experienced erotic transference requires substantial skill, and supervision may be necessary. How to work with the sexual transference during psychotherapy is a topic that transcends the scope of this chapter.

Relationship Between Sexual Fantasy and Sexual Activity

Sexual fantasy is experienced by postpubertal males in a pressured way that requires orgiastic discharge of sexual tension. As fate would have it, erotic sensation happens to be experienced most intensely during early adolescence before young men are legally allowed to drive, vote, serve in the military, or consume alcoholic beverages. Even so, many stumble toward imposing some degree of thoughtful delay between the experience of sexual desire and enactment of interpersonal sexual activity. Learning proceeds at a variable rate and may be especially impaired in men who have psychopathology associated with diminished impulse control. Men with diverse Axis I and II psychiatric disorders fall into this group.

Sexual Impulsivity and Compulsivity

One way of thinking about psychopathology involving sexuality is to conceptualize the relationships among sexual desire, sexual activity, ego functions, and the manifestations of conscience. Ideally sexual impulses are regulated by conscience and personality functions that include reality testing and judgment, so that neither antisocial nor self-destructive sexual activity is carried out. These constraints are violated by patients who have diverse psychiatric disorders. In assessing these patients it is helpful to keep a principle in mind concerning the relationship between psychotherapy and psychopharmacology. When erotic fantasies motivate maladaptive sexual activity in the presence of Axis I or Axis II psychiatric disorders, adequate treatment of the disorders must be carried out in addition to psychotherapeutic treatment that focuses on the patient's sexuality. It need hardly be emphasized that psychopharmacologic treatment is mandated for many disorders. We stress this in order to diminish the likelihood that underlying psychiatric disorders may be overlooked in some patients whose sexual experience and activity may be dramatic and vivid. As a general rule, psychotherapeutic progress in focal areas of functioning such as sexual experience and activity is enhanced when all the disorders affecting the individual are treated adequately.

Destructive Sexual Activity

Destructive sexual activity can be thought of as activity that is destructive to others or to the self. In both cases the individual's sexual activity may have a peremptory, pressured, driven, impulsive or compulsive quality. Countless instances of both types exist.

Hypersexuality is a well-known aspect of mania. Perhaps less well appreciated is that sexual fantasies experienced in a context of the increased arousal characteristic of hypomania and mixed manic or hypomanic-depressive affect may lead to diminished impulse control, impaired judgment, and precipitous sexual activity. This is a feature of many patients with atypical bipolar disorders and bipolar II disorder. In other patients, the affective combinations might differ. Destructive sexual activity may be motivated by sexual fantasies embedded in mixtures of feelings of erotic lust, anger, anxiety, irritability, or hostility, and in certain types of depression. The man experiences feelings of intense global arousal characterized by restlessness, an overwhelming pressured need to participate in the type of sexual activity that he fantasizes about, and sexual arousal.

Anxiety and hostility are usually mixed with erotic affect to some degree in all men during states of sexual arousal. The sexologist and psychoanalyst Robert Stoller (1979) even speculated that a certain amount of hostility was necessary in everyone in order for passionate sexual arousal to occur. The issue then is not whether other affects are present during sexual arousal but rather their unique intensities and the characteristics of the mixture. A crucial clinical issue concerns the person's *coping capacity*—in this case the capacity to tolerate the experience of intensely arousing affects that include lust, and their simultaneously occurring fantasies, without immediately attempting to translate the imagined scenarios into action. Patients with multiaxial difficulties such as mood disorders interacting with personality disorders are obviously at particular risk for repetitive destructive sexual activities. Substance abuse is frequently present as well.

In some individuals sexual fantasies are experienced in a particularly urgent way, virtually compelling action (Stoller 1975). The mandatory, driven quality of sexual activity in such persons has a compulsive quality: such patients have prominent obsessive-compulsive features. In recent years a movement has arisen to refer to patients who carry out repetitive destructive sexual activities as *sexual addicts.* Sexual addiction is not a DSM-IV diagnosis, and we see no reason for its usage. Sexual activities are not based on the physiologic characteristics that define addiction—tolerance, dependence, and the occurrence of withdrawal symptoms when the substance is not available (American Psychiatric Association 1994; Black 1998). Although their pleasurable qualities may be seen as analogous to those provided by drugs of abuse, our view is that the analogy goes only so far, and it does not add to a clear conceptual framework for understanding these patients. We find it helpful to understand the patient's sexual motivations within the context of a detailed diagnostic assessment of psychopathology, utilizing the multiaxial format of DSM-IV and a psychodynamically oriented developmental history. Treatment planning made on the basis of such assessment leads to different strategies for combining psychopharmacologic and psychotherapeutic management for different patients.

People who repetitively commit antisocial activities vary as to their dangerousness. Similarly, in the sexual arena the level of aggression experienced by the patient and expressed in the form of violence, whether sexual or otherwise, dictates the appropriate clinical response. Patients who enact antisocial, violent sexual fantasies are seen, as a general rule, in the criminal justice system, not in the outpatient practices of psychodynamically oriented psychotherapists. As is true of other nonviolent criminals, patients who carry out nonviolent but nonetheless antisocial and criminal sexual acts, such as exhibitionists or pedophiles, frequently receive treatment within the context of the criminal justice system. For those who require treatment outside of institutions, psychodynamically oriented psychotherapy in itself is not usually the treatment of choice—although some type of dynamic therapy may be part of a more inclusive treatment plan that includes medications and group and family therapies. This latter point is true of patients who meet criteria for paraphilias of diverse types. Such disorders are usually best treated with behavior therapy, social skills training, psychoeducation, pharmacotherapy, and family and group therapy, not individual psychodynamically oriented psychotherapy (Abel et al. 1992).

Sexual Guilt

In assessing the motivation of individuals to enact certain types of scenarios in an impulsive or compulsive manner, it is important to formulate the influence of guilt on the genesis of the patient's fantasy and its enactment. Consider the following vignette:

> Mr. C, a 50-year-old married man with bipolar II disorder and mixed personality disorder, presented for treatment of depression. In his history were episodes of impulsively seeking sex with

street prostitutes—and on more than one occasion of having been assaulted by their pimps or robbed. He fully realized the dangers of his activity. He was a successful professional who also frequented expensive houses of prostitution where the clientele was protected from abuse. Ever since his early teen years, Mr. C had recurrent erotic fantasies of having sex with street prostitutes. He was able to restrain the impulse to act on these fantasies much of the time, but when he felt, as he put it, "agitated," he succumbed. By agitated, he meant a dysphoric mood state consisting of increased irritability, anxiety, fleeting feelings of pessimistic depression, arousal, and decreased need for sleep. The particular pleasure he felt in enacting the fantasy of sex with a street prostitute was unique and difficult for him to describe precisely.

Diagnostic assessment of Mr. C's psychiatric disorders led to psychopharmacologic intervention. After he began a regimen of a mood stabilizer and a selective serotonin reuptake inhibitor, the specific scenario of his sexual fantasy life did not change, but his impulse control increased greatly. Mr. C then was able to use the psychotherapeutic situation to understand the origins and motivations of his sexual life. His developmental history revealed that the uniquely compelling quality of the prostitute fantasy was associated with a sense of risk (which Mr. C did not experience when he patronized the more affluent and secure brothels) and the likelihood of punishment. Mr. C, who had been raised as a devout believer in a religion that condemned premarital and extramarital sexuality, could simultaneously enact forbidden impulses and atone for them by placing himself at risk of being physically beaten and degraded.

The developmental features of Mr. C's psychosexual history were unique. But the more general pattern of a conflict between impulse and conscience—much of which occurs unconsciously and thus out of awareness—is an extremely common motivator of self-destructive sexual activity and occurs in patients with diverse mental disorders. As seen in Mr. C's history, guilt about sexuality sometimes takes the form of physically enacted self-abuse, in the service of atonement. The patient may engineer the social scenario so that the abuse is carried out by someone else, or he may carry it out by himself. Countless examples of the latter dynamic come readily to mind from the experience of clinicians who have worked with institutionalized patients. Wrist slashing, head-banging, cutting and wounding the surface of the body, attempted removal of the eyes, and autopenectomy are only some of the more extreme responses of psychotic patients (often under the influence of command hallucinations) to sexual impulses that they experience as incompatible with their consciences. Such patients often experience in an amplified fashion psychological conflicts that less disturbed patients express in a more subtle fashion.

Atonement by physical suffering, wounding, or suicidal behavior are part of the repertoire of self-destructive acts motivated by inappropriate responses of conscience. Consider the following vignette:

> Mr. D, a conscientious and highly moral middle-aged man, experienced in midlife the onset of intense recurrent voyeuristic urges that he felt were disgusting. Although he controlled his impulse to peep at women from his darkened apartment window using binoculars, he occasionally purchased pornographic videocassettes, which he viewed secretly while masturbating. His only sexual partner was his wife, and although the couple had sexual activity regularly, Mr. D experienced it as boring and repetitive. His feelings of passionate interest in his wife had long since abated, and each was chronically hostile, albeit in a somewhat disguised way, to the other. Mr. D sought psychotherapy for episodes that he labeled "alcoholism." These episodes were partially motivated by a desire to diminish the intensity of his sexual cravings and partially to atone for them. On a few occasions he became inappropriately inebriated in work-related social situations, with consequences that were quite destructive for his career.
>
> Psychotherapeutic exploration revealed a connection between Mr. D's unconscious desire to atone for unacceptable sexual impulses by punishing himself with vocational failures. His alcohol abuse was not primary and subsided rapidly in the presence of appropriate psychotherapeutic intervention and pharmacologic treatment. In Mr. D's case his unacceptable sexual fantasies were enacted only to a minimal degree. He denied his troubled relationship with his wife, and his intense pathologic enactment was in the service of his rigid conscience structure.

Boundary Violations

Self-destructive sexual activity is often enacted, not just imagined. Many types of boundary violations in vocational settings fall into this category, such as when teachers become sexually involved with students, administrators with their employees, military officers with enlisted personnel, and doctors and psychotherapists with their patients. We are not suggesting that isolated acts should be considered symptoms of specific types of psychopathology. Rather we believe that exploration of the underlying motives of patients who engage in these behaviors may reveal the need to be caught and punished as part of a motivational sequence associated with the enactment of sexual fantasies. Often the humiliation of being apprehended is experienced as punishment for the fantasies per se.

Undermining Love

The need for punishment is a common reason for undermining sexual love relationships. A person who feels the need to atone and be punished may sometimes do so by banishing himself from love. Extramarital relationships (and their equivalent among partners who are not married but may be monogamously committed) occur for many reasons and should not be considered inherently destructive or pathologic. However, self-destructiveness is often expressed in the context of such relationships and leads to exposure and to interpersonal chaos. Often pair bonds are ruptured, as are the extramarital affairs, and the cycle is repeated with other people as a consequence of pathology in the relationship between impulse and conscience.

The unconsciously motivated interdiction of sexual love may also take the form of loss of sexual desire within a love relationship that began as sexual or was on a developing sexual pathway. People with this type of difficulty often experience a form of what in psychodynamic jargon has been described as the "prostitute/madonna complex." The person experiences sexual arousal as inherently degrading; therefore, the person who he truly "loves" must be protected from his sexual passion. This problem occurs as a result of the individual's reaction to his sexual fantasies, which his rigid conscience interprets as taboo.

Freud: Moral Masochism and Sexual Masochism

Freud distinguished between moral and sexual masochism. By *moral masochism* he meant unconsciously motivated, repetitive self-destructive activity—so-called characterological masochism (Brenner 1959; Freud 1919/1955, 1924/1961; Glick and Myers 1988). *Sexual masochism,* in its most extreme form, refers to a specific type of paraphilia (American Psychiatric Association 1994). Fantasies of being humiliated, bound, punished, chastised, or even tortured are commonly experienced by men and women. These fantasies are not in themselves pathologic nor are their enactments, when engaged in with the flexibility characteristic of sexual experimentation or alternative forms of sexual expression. Such fantasies may express in a concrete and condensed way a drama depicting conflict between erotic experience and conscience. The feeling of being defiantly sexual and simultaneously being punished for it enhances sexual arousal for many people.

Internalized Homophobia

Self-destructiveness may also occur because of internalized homophobia in people whose conscience structures interdict homosexuality but whose sexual orientation is predominantly or exclusively homosexual. A particularly poignant form that this conflict sometimes takes is prolonged or even lifetime sexual celibacy. The person in such circumstances experiences homosexual fantasies that are unwanted and that recur despite the most extreme self-censure. Rather than translate these fantasies into actions, he avoids interpersonal sexual activity altogether, not only giving up the possibility of the pleasure of such activity but all possibility of finding sexual love. As painful as this conflict is, it is not inherently pathological. Sexual values may be embedded in larger religious or philosophical value systems, and in such instances, the person sacrifices sexual self-realization for goals that are experienced as higher. The conflict becomes pathological when the conscience or, in technical parlance, the superego functioning of the person operates in a rigid, maladaptive manner. There are no easily summarized guidelines for determining when this is the case, and gray zones certainly exist. The clinician is placed in the role of attempting to determine whether the patient's antihomosexual attitudes are manifestations of psychopathology. Sometimes these attitudes diminish when the identifications on which they are based are psychodynamically explored. Sometimes this does not occur, and the conflict turns out to be untreatable (Downey and Friedman 1995).

Although excessive inhibition of sexual activity may occur because of internalized homophobia, so may impulsive and compulsive sexual activity. People unconsciously motivated to atone for homosexual desire that they find unacceptable may participate in unsafe sexual practices in the same range of unwise or antisocial sexual activities as heterosexuals, engaging in sex with strangers who may harm them and placing themselves at risk of contracting HIV. Sometimes self-destructiveness is diminished as a result of a therapeutic stance that is "gay affirmative." Subgroups of patients exist who do not respond favorably to such an approach and who require exploratory psychotherapy (Friedman and Downey 1995a, 1995b, 1995c).

Special Clinical Problems in Men With Severe Personality Disorders

Men with severe personality disorders may experience many symptoms involving sexual fantasy and activity. For example, patients with narcissistic or antisocial personality disorders may be sexually exploitative of others, relating to them in a predatory, need-satisfying way. Space does not allow us to discuss the typical sexual pathology associated with each personality disorder. A particular issue that does warrant additional attention, however, is that of bisexuality and its relationship to disorders in which the sense of identity is weakened.

Men may be exclusively homosexual in orientation, exclusively heterosexual, or bisexual. Kinsey and co-workers noted that although most men experience exclusively heterosexual desires, many experienced some degree of bisexual fantasy during the course of their lives (Kinsey et al. 1948). Sexual orientation in itself is not indicative of psychopathology, and there is no evidence that men whose sexual fantasies are bisexual are more likely than gay or heterosexual men to experience mental disorders.

Bisexuality has probably been understudied in men because of homophobia and because our society offers no social niche for bisexual individuals. Clinical experience and anecdotal evidence indicate that bisexuality may be a stable, long-term trait. Some men enjoy bisexual lifestyles that are as fulfilling for them as heterosexual and gay lifestyles are for others. Like some heterosexual and gay patients, however, some bisexual men experience mental disorders. When these disorders are associated with a weakened sense of identity, a particular type of clinical problem often arises. Clinicians working with such patients are likely to be exposed to a request or demand expressed with pressured urgency to enable the patient to experience a unitary sense of identity over time. The patient attributes his difficulties to a single cause—uncertainty about being homosexual or heterosexual. The need for a rapid resolution to the sense of impaired identity is often couched in a simple question: "Am I gay or am I straight?" The patient conveys a sense that he attributes omnipotent power to the therapist and that if the therapist gives him the correct answer, his identity problems will be solved. Sadly this fails to happen.

Men with identity problems of this kind may or may not meet all of the DSM-IV criteria for borderline personality disorder (American Psychiatric Association 1994). From a somewhat less precise psychodynamic perspective, these patients may be conceptualized as having a borderline level of personality integration (Kernberg 1984). The patient is not borderline because he is bisexual, or bisexual because he is borderline. The two behavioral configurations co-occur by chance. These patients sometimes experience a need to place themselves into one of the two sexual orientation categories acceptable in our society, but neither heterosexual nor homosexual roles are possible for them. Accordingly they often alternate, first experiencing themselves as gay, then as straight, depending on their conscious and unconscious responses to interpersonal and vocational relationships and to the vicissitudes of daily life.

The clinician must avoid the trap—sometimes stumbled into by the inexperienced—of immediately siding with one or the other side of the patient's ambivalently experienced sexual orientations. An approach that is either overtly gay affirmative or overtly heterosexual affirmative is likely to fail and simply fuel the patient's feelings of inner chaos. Rather, the therapist should tolerate whatever anxieties are mobilized in himself or herself by the patient and nonjudgmentally and empathically explore the meaning of the patient's sexual fantasies in light of his history and total adaptation. Simultaneously, pharmacologic agents may be administered, if appropriate. Among the many issues that demand exploration are the degree to which the person is homophobic, the determinants of his conscience structure, the degree to which individuals in his social surroundings are heterosexist or homophobic, his religious and moral values, his cultural and subcultural roots, the nature of present life stresses that are of an immediately sexual nature, and also those that are not.

Sexual Orientation Conversion

The area of sexual orientation conversion is highly controversial because of its ideological, sociopolitical, religious, and ethical dimensions. It is important to distinguish between descriptive and prescriptive frames of reference in thinking about it clinically. Because heterosexuality is positively valued in our society by numerous religious and subcultural groups and homosexuality is negatively valued, almost all people who seek sexual orientation conversion experience themselves as homosexual and seek to become heterosexual.

To the degree that homosexual fantasies have been exclusive and enduring, they are not likely to be extinguished by any interpersonal, psychological, or religious intervention, no matter how intensely the patient seeks this intervention. Much publicity has been given to the fact that many alleged "homosexuals" have appeared to become transformed into "heterosexuals" through one intervention or another. Careful scrutiny of the available data indicates that when this occurs homosexual fantasies persist but are coped with differently than before. It is important to stress that many people who consider themselves heterosexual or wish to be so have histories of erotic fantasies that are bisexual (Nicolosi 1991). They may need therapeutic assistance in order not to attribute to these fantasies undue significance for their sense of identity.

In assessing patients who seek sexual orientation change, it is important for the clinician to conceptualize the origins and meanings of a person's antihomosexual value system. Is it primarily based on religious or moral values that anchor the patient's sense of identity, or is it a pathologic manifestation of internalized homophobia? We believe that once adequate assessment has been made, the crucial issue is informed consent. The patient must be made aware of realistic options from a descriptive perspective to whatever degree this is possible. The therapist should not attempt to impose a moral attitude about homosexuality on his or her patients. When patients seek to become part of the heterosexual mainstream with regard to social role and cultural participation, our view is that it is the therapist's responsibility to help them achieve this end. The therapist should not, however, prescribe this solution blindly without carrying out a meticulous assessment of the many parameters required to understand what appears to be an unambiguous manifest wish.

Conclusion

Human sexuality tends to be neglected by modern mental health clinicians. Because the regulation of self-esteem, the capacity to experience pleasure, and other important dimensions of functioning are intimately associated with sexual experience and activity, a sexual history should be a routine part of patient assessment. The range of sexual fantasies experienced by men is broad. Every type of image and situation depicted in fiction, including pornographic fiction and film, may be a scenario for male sexual fantasy. Freud's comments about so-called "perverse" desires aptly illustrate this point. In Freud's words:

Everyday experience has shown that most of these extensions (eg perversions), or at any rate the less severe of them, are constituents which are rarely absent from the sexual life of healthy people, and are judged by them no differently from other intimate events. If circumstances favour such an occurrence, normal people too can substitute a perversion of this kind for the normal sexual aim for quite a time, or can find place for the one alongside the other. No healthy person, it appears, can fail to make some addition that might be called perverse to the normal sexual aim; and the universality of this finding is in itself enough to show how inappropriate it is to use the word perversion as a term of reproach. (Freud 1905/1962, p. 51)

Because both sexual fantasy and activity are often experienced as shameful, patients may not spontaneously discuss their sexuality but are often relieved when therapists appropriately encourage them to do so. Sexual desires are or have been a crucial part of the inner life of all men. For those in whom sexual fantasies have diminished as a result of illness or treatment for illness, the deficit experienced by the self is always meaningful. This is often associated with impaired self-esteem and diminished engagement in life itself. The modern care-delivery ethic is focused on symptom relief and cost containment. Understanding and offering treatment to the men who happen to be psychotherapy patients require a broader framework, including awareness of the many meanings of their sexual lives.

References

Abel GG, Osborn C, Anthony D, et al: Current treatments of paraphiliacs. Annual Review of Sex Research 2:255–291, 1992

American Psychiatric Association: Diagnostic and Statistical Manual of Mental Disorders, 4th Edition. Washington, DC, American Psychiatric Association, 1994

Billy JO, Tanfer K, Grady WR, et al: The sexual behavior of men in the United States. Fam Plann Perspect 25:52–60, 1993

Black DW: Compulsive sexual behavior: a review. Journal of Practical Psychiatry and Behavioral Health 4:219–229, 1998

Blumstein P, Schwartz P: American Couples: Money, Work, Sex. New York, William Morrow, 1983

Bradford JMW, Greenberg DM: Pharmacological treatment of deviant sexual behavior. Annual Review of Sex Research 7:283–306, 1996

Brenner C: The masochistic character: genesis and treatment. J Am Psychoanal Assoc 7:197–226, 1959

Downey JI, Friedman RC: Internalized homophobia in lesbian relationships. J Am Acad Psychoanal 23:435–447, 1995

Freud S: The aetiology of hysteria (1896), in the Standard Edition of the Complete Psychological Works of Sigmund Freud, Vol 3. Translated and edited by Strachey J. London, Hogarth Press, 1962, pp 187–221

Freud S: The interpretation of dreams (1900), in the Standard Edition of the Complete Psychological Works of Sigmund Freud, Vols 4 and 5. Translated and edited by Strachey J. London, Hogarth Press, 1953

Freud S: Three Essays on the Theory of Sexuality (1905). New York, Avon Books, 1962

Freud S: Creative writers and daydreaming (1907), in The Freud Reader. Edited by Gay P. New York, WW Norton, 1989, pp 436–443

Freud S: A child is being beaten: a contribution to the study of the origins of sexual perversion (1919), in the Standard Edition of the Complete Psychological Works of Sigmund Freud, Vol 17. Translated and edited by Strachey J. London, Hogarth Press, 1955, pp 177–204

Freud S: The economic problem of masochism (1924), in the Standard Edition of the Complete Psychological Works of Sigmund Freud, Vol 19. Translated and edited by Strachey J. London, Hogarth Press, 1961, pp 157–179

Freund K, Langevin R, Chamberlayne R, et al: The phobic theory of male homosexuality. Arch Gen Psychiatry 31:495–499, 1974

Friedman RC: Male Homosexuality: A Contemporary Psychoanalytic Perspective. New Haven, CT, Yale University Press, 1988

Friedman RC: Internalized homophobia, pathological grief and high risk sexual behavior in a gay man with multiple psychiatric disorders. Journal of Sex Education and Therapy 23:115–120, 1998

Friedman RC, Downey JI: Homosexuality: special article. N Engl J Med 331:923–930, 1994

Friedman RC, Downey J: Biology and the Oedipus Complex. Psychoanal Q 64:234–265, 1995a

Friedman RC, Downey JI: Internalized homophobia and the negative therapeutic reaction. J Am Acad Psychoanal 23:99–113, 1995b

Friedman RC, Downey JI: MacIntosh study faulted (letter). J Am Psychoanal Assoc 43:304–305, 1995c

Friedman RC, Bucci W, Christian C, et al: Private psychotherapy patients of psychiatrist-psychoanalysts. Am J Psychiatry 155:1772–1774, 1998

Glick RA, Myers DI: Masochism: Current Psychoanalytic Perspectives. Hillsdale, NJ, Analytic Press, 1988

Hatfield E, Rapson RL: Historical and cross-cultural perspectives on passionate love and sexual desire. Annual Review of Sex Research 4:67–99, 1993

Isay R: Being Homosexual. New York, Farrar Straus Giroux, 1989

Isay RA: Becoming Gay. New York, Pantheon, 1996

Kernberg O: Object Relations Theory and Clinical Psychoanalysis. New York, Jason Aronson, 1976

Kernberg O: Severe Personality Disorders. New Haven, CT, Yale University Press, 1984

Kernberg O: Love Relations: Normality and Pathology. New Haven, CT, Yale University Press, 1995

Kinsey AC, Pomeroy WB, Martin CE: Sexual Behavior in the Human Male. Philadelphia, PA, WB Saunders, 1948

Laan E, Everaerd W: Determinants of female sexual arousal: psychophysiological theory and data. Annual Review of Sex Research 6:32–77, 1995

Lazar SG (ed): Extended dynamic psychotherapy: making the case in an era of managed care. Psychoanalytic Inquiry (suppl), 1997

Masters WH, Johnson VE: Human Sexual Response. Boston, MA, Little, Brown, 1966

McClintock M, Herdt G: Rethinking puberty: the development of sexual attraction. Current Directions in Psychological Science 5:167–183, 1996

Money J: Gay, Straight and In-Between. Oxford, England, Oxford University Press, 1988

Money J, Ehrhardt A: Man and Woman: Boy and Girl. Baltimore, MD, Johns Hopkins University Press, 1972

Moore B, Fine BD (eds): Psychoanalysis: The Major Concepts. New Haven, CT, Yale University Press, 1995

Nicolosi J: Reparative Therapy: Male Homosexuality. Northvale, NJ, Jason Aronson, 1991

Olds DD: Connectionism and psychoanalysis. J Am Psychoanal Assoc 42:581–613, 1994

Paredes RG, Baum MJ: Role of the medial preoptic area/anterior hypothalamus in the control of masculine sexual behavior. Annual Review of Sex Research 8:68–102, 1997

Person E: Dreams of Love and Fateful Encounters: The Power of Romantic Passion. New York, WW Norton, 1988

Person E: By Force of Fantasy. New York, Basic Books, 1995

Rosen RC, Beck JG: Patterns of Sexual Arousal: Psychophysiological Processes and Clinical Applications. New York, Guilford, 1988

Rosen RC, Leiblum SR: Erectile Disorders: Assessment and Treatment. New York, Guilford, 1992

Seidman SN, Rieder RO: A review of sexual behavior in the United States. Am J Psychiatry 151:330–341, 1994

Stoller R: Pornography and perversion, in Perversion: The Erotic Form of Hatred. London, Karnac, 1975, pp 63–92

Stoller R: Sexual Excitement: Dynamics of Erotic Life. New York, Pantheon, 1979

Tyson P: Theories of female psychology. J Am Psychoanal Assoc 42:447–469, 1994

Ursano RJ, Sonneberg SM, Lazar SG: Psychodynamic Psychotherapy: Principles and Techniques in the Era of Managed Care. Washington, DC, American Psychiatric Press, 1998

Chapter 2

Male Heterosexuality

Stephen B. Levine, M.D.

Heterosexuality, the sexual orientation of over 90% of American men (Billy et al. 1993), can be considered to be a line of psychological development. Heterosexuality begins to evolve emotionally and cognitively in childhood using the boy's genetically programmed capacity for sexual response (Martinson 1980). Heterosexuality continues to be refined throughout adolescence and most of adulthood. At various stages of life, a man's heterosexuality can be well managed into personal and partner psychological health or poorly managed into personal and partner despair. Heterosexuality is therefore a continuing developmental challenge. Male heterosexuality can be defined as an evolving mental organization that directs the sexual and romantic interests and behaviors of males toward females for the vast majority of their life span.

How any orientation—heterosexuality, bisexuality, homosexuality, or uncertain—comes about remains a partial scientific mystery. Discussions usually focus on the relative roles of biology, family dynamics, and social learning; however, the question is almost exclusively addressed only for homosexuality (Sell 1997). Although the origins of homosexuality continue to generate many politically sensitive discussions, no replicated data set has answered the question with ringing clarity (Pillard and Bailey 1995). The comparable question about heterosexuality has never generated research, perhaps because it is assumed to be simultaneously biologically, dynamically, and socially programmed. Science has not provided a verified mechanism of development to explain how heterosexuality comes into being and how it evolves.

In this chapter, I descriptively address four questions about heterosexuality:

1. What are the developmental potentials of heterosexuality?
2. What skills seem to be necessary to reach these potentials?
3. What are the usual clinical signs of failure to attain these potentials?
4. What problematic subtypes of heterosexuality can be defined?

The Evolution of Heterosexuality

Proto-heterosexuality

The ordinary pathway of heterosexual development begins with a proto-heterosexual form prior to puberty. Its earliest conspicuous forerunner is often the formation of a boyish masculinity during the preschool years. During the school years, proto-heterosexuality is generally recognized by the boy's identifications with boys and men. Some sets of behaviors are socially gender-conforming—that is, recognized as boyish or, if not typical, accepted by the family as masculine (e.g., being a violinist disinterested in sports). At this age, many gender-typical boys display a feigned disinterest in girls, have vocal displays of disgust over adult heterosexual displays of affection, and engage in limited masturbation (orgasm usually does not occur until puberty). No one set of characteristics, however, invariably predicts adolescent heterosexuality or the inevitability of developing another orientation (Green 1987).

Adolescent Heterosexuality

Heterosexuality undergoes a dramatic lasting change as a result of two stages of androgen production: adrenarche and gonadarche (McClintock and Herdt 1996). By adolescence, androgens create a mental state dominated by sexually arousing images of the female form, their hidden body parts, and their immediate cloth coverings and an intense increased cathexis of the penis and a preoccupation with its function. Adolescent boys consciously manage the subjective effects of this state through masturbation. The behavioral effects of this state are managed through increasing social skills, which lead to sexual behaviors with consenting partners and deepening functional appreciation of the complexity of intimate relationships. Peers are aware of the recurring sexual excitement experienced by teenage males. Its presence is often obvious to junior and senior high school teachers, who frequently make references to their male students' hormones. Sons try to prevent their parents from knowing about their eroticized minds, but of course parents—particularly fathers—are cognizant of the sexual excitement experienced by adolescents. Parents—much to their sons' relief—often pretend that they do not see.

Adult Heterosexuality

From this sexualized teenage beginning, the next momentous developmental landmark of heterosexuality is the ability to affectionately and physically love an individual woman. This process takes years and has many stops along the way. Many men think that they are in love only to discover that they were mistaken (Levine 1998a). During these courtships, many men come to realize that their search for a partner is affected profoundly by how they privately view their looks, capabilities, and vocational prospects. Once the woman is identified and the man both declares and acts like he is willing and able to comply with the many requirements of a loving relationship, he positions himself to begin the next and the major heterosexual challenge: to abide with his partner as they go through life together. If finding the right woman to be one's partner is considered to be a difficult process, abiding with her through long periods of mutual development must be considered far more challenging and arduous.

The Final Accomplishment

The final, paramount developmental landmark of heterosexuality is the emergence of a genuine nonsexual appreciation of the capacities, roles, and styles inherent in women's lives. It is the ability to see beyond an individual woman to women in general; to appreciate and respect the important differences in their capacities, roles, and styles; and to make judgments about them on matters other than their physical appeal. The developmental task involves routinely exercising respectful judgments about individual women and understanding their psychology. Until this task is genuinely accomplished, men—who know the unstated rules of social life—often simply act the part. Although each accomplishment (i.e., loving, abiding, and appreciating) has roots in earlier developmental processes, each is likely to be epigenetic—that is, loving an individual woman arrives first, a deep appreciation of women in general comes last.

Rephrasing the Developmental Challenge of Heterosexuality

Whatever the social, sexual, reproductive, and psychological concerns of heterosexual males may be at any given time, their ultimate sexual challenge is to maintain a supportive relationship to their partners. The challenge is to be a positive rather than a destructive force in women's lives so as not to reduce a partner's mental state to lasting rage and despair.

From male child, to gradually emancipated adolescent, to young adult searching for a life-mate while developing social skills and refined judgment, to adult struggling to integrate sexual, marital, social, economic, psychological, and parental demands, to an older man trying to maintain his dignity in the face of his losses, the male heterosexual life cycle contains countless inconspicuous transformations (Erickson 1963). In terms of developmental potential, these transformations are challenges to men to quickly, consistently, and progressively become non-exploitative in relationship to women. Men are slow to understand this because exploiting women for sexual gratification is culturally celebrated as an epitome of early adult masculinity. What a man does with his heterosexuality partly enables and partly reflects his maturation.

Default Heterosexuality

What Heterosexual Men Have in Common

The adolescent heterosexual experience is never completely erased from consciousness. The ability to be erotically aroused by images of women's anatomy, sexual behavior, and excitement remains in privacy as a healthy subjective capacity. This capacity is now defined as *default heterosexuality*. In order to realize his maturational potentials and remain healthy, a man must over-lay—not obliterate—the default eroticization of women's bodies and the promise of its sexual pleasures with the more complex and sophisticated abilities to love, abide, and appreciate women. About the only thing that heterosexual men have in common with one another is their basic appreciation of and gravitation to-ward attractive (however defined) women and their body parts.

This basic commonality is associated with an erotic imagina-tion of women as a promised source of physical and psychologi-cal pleasure. Men in groups tend to elicit each other's default heterosexuality and often rate, in some manner, women's beauty or sex appeal. When alone in the company of women, men are generally able to suppress their default patterns and focus on matters beyond the body, but breakthroughs, particularly via hu-mor, are common.

What Makes Heterosexuals Different From One Another?

The vast diversity among heterosexual men of any particular age group is created by their achievements in getting beyond private mental domination by their default sexual responses. In adoles-cence and young adulthood, this may be related to differences in the strength of their biological sexual drives; their inherent ag-gression toward women; the civilizing effect of their maternal, paternal, and sibling relationships; their basic mental health; the influence of their school and religious experiences; and their identifications with role models. These factors participate in the formation of the conscience, which will regulate the behavioral expression of sexual attractions for most of the remainder of adulthood.

We do not expect heterosexual adolescents to be able to en-tirely, calmly, and smoothly control their basic sexual excitements when alone with adolescent girls. Subjective and social awk-wardness is expected. We do expect them to control themselves within certain standards, however. Such internal subjective and external behavioral development takes much time. The process is a subtle one filled with steps forward and steps backward, and it is assisted greatly by societal demands to be mature and by opportunities to get to know women as people.

Heterosexual men also differ in their relationship to their own erotic imagination. For some men it is an inner sexual aesthetic standard that quietly leads their search for a mate—"I want a wife who has legs that never quit!" For some it is simply an arena in which the sexual contexts that excite are staged—"Well, I dated her, so I thought about her body." For others, it is a grandiose retreat where the man assumes mythic proportions—"There I am irresistible—a James Bond." Men do not give equal credence to their erotic imaginations. Some use it to define themselves—"Sex is my essence; I am a cocksman." Most men are less intense—"Sure sex is important, but so are a lot of other things." Many men are uncertain what to do with and think about their default heterosexuality; others are clear: they consider it a sin.

The Potentials Are Quite Difficult to Attain

Like nonsexual adult developmental tasks (Erickson 1963), attaining and maintaining heterosexuality's lofty potentials are extremely difficult to attain efficiently. Men spend years in pursuit of these goals. Two aspects of reality often delay or derail them. First, it is often privately difficult to know who women are in terms of their personhood apart from their sexual appeal. Men must struggle to override their sexual preoccupations to learn about the woman as a person. In this sense, default heterosexuality might be labeled a maturational obstacle, a prejudice, a large blind spot, or if one has a sense of humor . . . a disease. Second, whereas socialization exposes the man to the discovery that women are far more complex than they previously imagined ("Boy! I was naive!"), courtship exposes men to their fear, disappointment, and anger over rejection. Whether imagined or experienced, rejection can generate hidden anger toward women. This anger adds to whatever inherent aggressive tendencies already existed. Loving in an abiding manner depends on the man's ability to neutralize this aggression toward women based on his experiences with rejection throughout his life. Experiences with personal abuse, neglect, injustice, and abandonment make such neutralization more difficult to attain.

In successfully modifying the power of their default heterosexuality, men improve their reality testing and remain informed by their inner erotic responses but not personally or socially dominated by them. In surviving rejections, men learn (through their private vulnerability) that women have a comparable inner vulnerability. This enables them to be more considerate.

The Infrastructure of Heterosexuality

Clinicians may recognize unhealthy heterosexuality by the presence of persistent unusual erotic preoccupations. These fantasies involve images of being a woman or various paraphiliac themes. Men with ordinary default heterosexuality have a better disguised infrastructure. They have occasional erotic fantasies, curiosities, attractions, and dreams that suggest that there is more within the ordinary default orientation than can immediately be appreciated from its surface manifestations (Stoller 1975). Ascertaining the contents of the hidden dynamic infrastructure of default heterosexuality, however, is a matter of speculation.

Here is one possibility: Ordinary heterosexual male eroticism contains many impulses whose verbal or behavioral expression to most women would immediately create alarm. One theme of such impulses is the idea of being in charge. Embedded in the infrastructure is an aspiration for a power inequity. Heterosexual men have a subtle aspiration for domination of the partner, the ability to sexually command and be obeyed and the capacity to control and make the woman do the man's sexual bidding—all within reasonable limits.

The aspiration for a power inequity is seen more clearly in some heterosexual men with sadomasochism (Weinberg 1994). Their intensely arousing sexual scripts grossly but concretely exaggerate prosaic heterosexual themes. Their ritualized dominant behavior seems to be an attempt to reduce the rich complexity of male-female sexual relationships to one simplified notion of the essence of masculinity and femininity: "I, the man, am the natural commander; and you, the woman, are the natural follower."

For sadomasochism or any unusual aspect of sexual identity (Levine 1988) to be used as a source of illumination of ordinary heterosexuality, however, one has to assume that the default structure is a developmental accomplishment, that it is formed by the mastery of childhood developmental sequences (Freud 1905/1971). With this assumption, one might use transvestic fetishism to argue that default structure contains a hidden feminine identification. Fetishists feel compelled to act out their feminine identification and envy; the "femininity" of men with an ordinary default structure does not intrude on and limit their sexual behavior. The diversity of adult sexual developmental outcomes in the population is impressive. Many investigators have thought that this variety begins with a fundamental bisexual potential of all humans (Stoller 1972). Such speculations, correct or not, point to the presence of a dynamic, partially conscious infrastructure.

The Concept of Male Heterosexual Developmental Failure

The Source of Heterosexual Men's Mental Suffering

Men suffer from their failures to love, abide, and appreciate women. Mental health professionals rarely discuss their male heterosexual patients in these terms, however. Instead, we concentrate on the consequences of these failures: depression, anxiety, substance abuse, addictions, and even psychosis. An increasingly common problem with our modern approach is that in focusing on these symptomatic patterns we often are blind to the developmental failures that played a major role in creating them. Modern psychiatry, in its romance with the brain's anatomic and biochemical dimensions, has moved away from the idea that psychiatric diagnoses have anything to do with psychological development and love (Lewis 1998). In this chapter, I make the opposite assumption: psychiatric illnesses and undiagnosed emotional decompensations can be the direct consequences of adult developmental failures and not merely the sources of those failures. This assumption becomes more compelling when clinicians understand the complexity of sexual desire.

The Tripartite Nature of Sexual Desire

Caution! Clinicians often oversimplify the concept of sexual desire in four ways:

- We often speak of sexual desire as if it is a singular, biologically determined phenomenon (Kaplan 1995). Sexual desire is manifested by erotic thoughts and dreams, sensitivity to sexual stimuli in the environment, heightened arousal to sexual stimuli, planning for orgasm, initiation of masturbation or partner sexual behavior, and receptivity to partner sexual initiations. Sometimes all of this is reduced to an answer on a questionnaire about "interest in sex" that is rated on a scale from 1 to 5 (Goldstein et al. 1998). Clinicians often miss the fact that men's sexual desire is also psychologically and socially driven.
- We authoritatively interchange four words for sexual desire—libido, drive, interest, and desire. Sexual desire is an amalgamation of separate biological, psychological, and social forces. Although each of these separate forces may work in concert, they are often in conflict with one another.
- We act as though desire is distinctly different from the process of sexual arousal. We currently think of it as the first step of sexual function, as that phenomenon that precedes arousal. Sexual desire is often indistinguishable from early sexual arousal, a physiologic state manifested by increased penile blood flow, volume, and sensations. Sexual desire may well be only the brain's sexual arousal capacities activated by endogenous neurochemistry, environmental sexual stimuli, or a promising social context (Janssen and Everaerd 1993).
- We fail to appreciate that men's accounts of their sexual desire are often grossly inaccurate. Their accounts are shaped by who asks the questions, their notion of what other men expe-

rience, and their facility at recognizing and labeling certain experiences as sexual. Men actually experience desire for sex in four important ways:

- In a quantitatively variable but reasonably regular buildup of sexual tensions
- In response to reading about or seeing the sexual activity of others
- In hoped-for anticipation of sexual behavior within their relationships with partners
- In response to alcohol and other readily abusable substances

Young and middle-aged men tend to represent themselves as existing in a tonic state of desire. Older men freely state that their sexual desire is occasional. Some men acknowledge that it is more pride than drive.

Biological Component of Desire—Sexual Drive

The strength and the frequency of sexual urges are typically stronger in the 15 years following puberty than at any other time in a man's life. This means that the body's most sexually efficient era is youth. It is then when men have the quickest ejaculations, shortest refractory periods, and highest masturbatory frequencies. The neuroendocrine physiology that accounts for the sexual characteristics of youth and for the general decline in drive as men age is not well understood. In lower animals, the hypothalamic anteromedial preoptic area contains nuclei that are referred to as the sexual drive center. This area can be manipulated pharmacologically and stereotactically to enhance and inhibit sexual behavior (Hines and Collaer 1993). In humans, nuclei adjacent to the third ventricle have been shown to be relevant to interest in sexual behavior, but various other sites in the central nervous system (particularly in the limbic system) and neurotransmitter systems (particularly dopaminergic systems) are also thought to be involved (Melis et al. 1987). Only a small amount of androgen is necessary to optimize male sexual function. This information does not amount to a sophisticated physiologic grasp of sexual drive and arousal as they normally evolve during the life cycle; such information does not yet exist.

What is empirically known with far greater certainty is the capacity of medications to dampen sexual drive and arousal mechanisms. Chief among these medications are the selective serotonin reuptake inhibitors (SSRIs)—fluoxetine, paroxetine, sertraline, and fluvoxamine. The SSRIs are more similar than different in terms of their sexual effects. They most conspicuously limit orgasmic attainment in approximately 60% of patients, create separate sexual desire complaints in an additional 15% of patients, and lead an unknown percentage of patients to switch or stop their medications (Montejo-Gonzalez et al. 1997). Each patient has to balance the benefits of the drug with its sexual consequences, most of which are negative. Antihypertensive agents, opioids, anticonvulsants, and phenothiazines also take their toll. Less commonly used agents that lower testosterone levels (e.g., estrogens, progesterone) or those that raise estrogen levels (e.g., digitalis, spironolactone, cimetidine) adversely influence drive and arousal. Despite the public's endless search for an aphrodisiac, substances of abuse in the long term are generally more subtly destructive than enhancing of sexual life. The medical profession does not have a medication that reliably enhances sexual drive, despite our many prescriptions of trazodone, yohimbine, testosterone, methylphenidate, and bupropion (Rosen and Ashton 1993). The extent to which drugs affect a patient depends on the patient's age, disease status, and previous sexual capacity. Middle-aged and older men are expected to have more noticeable drive reductions on these medications because their drive and arousal mechanisms are already less efficient (Rowland et al. 1993).

Psychological Component of Desire—Sexual Motive

The common observation that some men with a receptive sexual partner prefer frequent masturbation and avoid sex with their partner is one reason to emphasize that drive is not synonymous with desire. A man must be willing to have sex with a particular woman.

Many nonbiological factors account for a man's willingness or unwillingness to have sex. The acquisition of social skills; increasing grasp of the personhood of a partner; the ability to identify, accept, and resolve interpersonal conflict; and the capacity to trust and remain trustworthy are a few factors that affect the frequency and quality of partner sexual interaction. The fact that many partnerships are asexual while the two individuals are not also reminds us that the clinician must be able to reliably separate drive from motive in the consulting room.

Men often persist in the illusion that their sexual interest is relatively stable because it is less context driven than is their partner's sexual desire. Women's sexual drives and motives are highly context driven. As men live with healthy women and watch their drive manifestations vary with the menstrual cycle, pregnancy, lactation, medications, perimenopause, and menopause, and as they observe how the fluctuations in the amount and quality of time spent with the partner and the children affect women's willingness to behave sexually, they conclude that their own sexual desire is a constant. But it is not. It is only that their sexual drive is typically higher. (The mean testosterone level in men is 500 µg/dl whereas that of women is 38 µg/dl; in both sexes there is a poor correlation between testosterone level and sexual drive manifestations.) Many hypoactive sexual desire disorders in heterosexual men are due to marital dilemmas that the men had a major role in constructing (Levine 1998c; Polonsky 1998).

Men's motives are also context driven. For example, in couples who have long-lasting, satisfying sexual partnerships, serious illness in the woman may eventually eradicate the man's motive to make love. Sexual willingness to make love involves a perception of the partner as reasonably healthy. Her worsening multiple sclerosis, cancer, Alzheimer's disease, emphysema, schizophrenia, and so on at some unique level of severity will rob the man of his willingness to make love. Within this context, his drive manifestations may persist, although he may not share this fact with his physician until he is reassured that the doctor will not think less of him. The man's sexual sensibilities are eventually exceeded by illness severity—"Well, she is too sick now." He becomes unwilling to make love with his partner, even if she requests it.

Depression and other individual states of psychopathology may be considered as an important individual context through which to consider sexual motives. When anhedonia, pessimism, distrust, lack of confidence, indecision, and other symptoms dominate men's mental lives, their anticipation of and experience of sexual behavior may alter their reports of their drive, motive, or desire—"I still feel the urge, but I figure, why bother?" Classic teachings about depression often stress that "libido" is diminished with depression, but careful study in a clinic specializing in depression has suggested that this may not be the case in all seriously depressed men (Nofzinger et al. 1993). Anhedonia dominates the recognition and reporting of drive and dampens motive. Clinical work with paraphiliac men, however, has generated the opposite impression (Kafka 1997). Depression can be coped with and defended against by increasing sexual expression. It is less certain whether to label the compulsive sexual behaviors of hypersexual patients as increased drive or increased motivation.

Social Component of Desire—Sexual Wish

Men learn about sex and form sexual expectations from their culture. Cultural influence begins with the family of origin and gradually expands outward to other social sources of learning. These sources must be subtle and involve identifying social context clues and defining personal internal standards for civilized sexual behaviors. All social sources are related in some way to conscience, which is lurking within men's motives and wishes.

The frequency with which a man requests sexual behavior within a relationship may depend on his notions of how often it is normal for a man of his age to have sex. If he learns that it is every day, his negotiations for frequency of sex will be quite different than if he learns that it is weekly. The differing ages at which partner sex is first experienced (later in orthodox religious communities) and the varying rates of partner sexual behavior in different subcultures (more frequent adolescent sex in poor cultures in the United States) reflect the influence of social organizations on sexual expression.

The man's wish for sex is a vital component to consider in the clinical setting because many older men who seek help for erectile dysfunction say that their desire is "normal," meaning only that they *want* to have sex again (Levine 1992). Their drives may be absent, and although they have a receptive sexual partner, they may not have had any physical contact for years. They are speaking of the wish component of sexual desire. The unwary clinician who equates drive, desire, interest, and libido may hear that the patient's libido is normal and may not understand the patient's resistance to treatment.

Summary of Sexual Desire

Sexual desire is the complex, ever-evolving byproduct of the interaction of drive, motive, and wish. The conscience controls the behavioral expressions of sexual desire. It is a mark of a mature man to be able to negotiate for the satisfaction of his sexual excitements within a context that is acceptable to him and his partner. Many men who lack sexual motive for their partners have lively drive and wish components. Many men without drive have persistent wishes to behave sexually. All sexual dysfunctions—even those that present as problems with erections, ejaculation, or pain—have important relationships to the man's sexual drive, motive, and wish. These in turn reflect the underlying accomplishments or lack thereof of the heterosexual developmental potentials.

Common Manifestations of Heterosexual Developmental Failures

The Problem With Conceptualizing Heterosexual Patterns

The developmental demands of being a heterosexual man generate a wide array of personal and social difficulties. Although clinicians routinely encounter these difficulties, we rarely conceptualize them as having any causal relationship to heterosexuality per se. We may casually account for them with concepts that resemble diagnoses—for example, he . . . is depressed, drinks too much, is neurotic, is a bit crazy, has a personality disorder, and so on. Our language rarely reflects an understanding that the difficulty is a consequence of the man's prior choices, his thinking, his pattern of regulating his sexual attractions, or, most important, his style of being heterosexual.

A Caveat

These perils of adult development have affected so many people that many readers will consider their mere enunciation to be politically insensitive, moralistic, ill-informed, or socially incorrect. Some may be infuriated because the designated patterns seem to confuse differing social values (e.g., "People have a right to be unfaithful.") and personal choices (e.g., "I decided not to tell my partner about my unwillingness to have a child.") with developmental pitfalls (e.g., failure to work through maternal neglect). Others may think that I am advocating a personal value system that naively states that men should be honest; marry and live with their wives forever; and strive to conduct their sexual lives in a manner that goes against many widespread cultural patterns of male entitlement to sexual freedom. In contrast, I think I am pointing out the ways in which men commonly mismanage their heterosexual desires and adversely influence their own and their family's emotional lives. I think of some of these patterns as problematic subtypes of heterosexuality. I leave the ultimate judgment to the reader.

The heuristic value of these patterns lies in their ability to expand our appreciation of heterosexual developmental failures, not in their ability to generate DSM-IV diagnoses. The complexity of any heterosexual relationship exceeds most points on this list because two personalities and a culture create the relationship. This list is only an attempt to focus on the man's subtle contributions to his life problems.

The Patterns

- **Aggressive sexual behaviors.** These men have not progressed developmentally very far from their dominating and often paraphiliac default heterosexuality. Sexualized aggression has both criminal and noncriminal forms:

- Serious criminal episodes (e.g., rape, incest, stalking)
- Less serious criminal episodes (e.g., exhibitionism, obscene phone calling, voyeurism, frotteurism)
- Fantasy preoccupation with these same activities without behavioral expression
- Rough sex that often causes pain or injury to sexual partner

- **Patterns that keep men from sexual relationships with women as people:**

  - Fixation on erotic imagery—men whose otherwise conventional erotic interests are gratified by pornography, strip shows, or Internet contacts.
  - Profound subjective fears—men who are unable to socialize with women in a dating context. Their shyness renders them dependent on masturbation, prostitution, or partner encounters only while intoxicated.
  - Profound social deficits—men who recurrently fail to realistically gauge the intangibles and unstated aspects of dating. These men long remain unaware of their social unattractiveness because of their insensitivity to women or their sexual eagerness.

- **Patterns of duplicity that keep men from being known by partners:**

  - Don Juanism—preoccupation with seduction as the realization of the pinnacle of masculinity. The risk that these sexually active, potent men face is the inability to feel affection for any woman whom he can sexually enjoy and the inability to sexually enjoy any woman for whom he feels affection. When these men marry, they are prone to create an asexual marriage that is quickly characterized by infidelity.

- Extreme emphasis on youth, beauty, or both, which relegates all other aspects of the partner to a subordinate position.
- An unwillingness to be faithful. This can range from a single episode of partner deception to "womanizing." Even a single episode, particularly when a new love relationship is involved, eradicates the man's ability to be spontaneous and honest; it can undermine his marriage even when his wife is unaware of his infidelity. Repeated infidelity not only tends to destroy the fabric of marriage and family life but renders the partner chronically humiliated, demeaned, and enraged.

- **Patterns of failure to adjust to the needs of the partner,** which generate alienation:

  - Based on the man's inflexible insistence on his way in most matters—that is, his interpretation of how to be a "man" in a marriage.
  - Based on the man's inability to understand and accommodate to the woman's patterns and sensibilities—"Women are from a different planet!"
  - Based on his perception that he is recurrently the victim of the woman's controlling nature.
  - Based on the woman's lack of emotional satisfaction from sex because of the man's sexual patterns.
  - Based on his unsubtle disinterest in his children.

- Egregious narcissism that leads to failures in the sphere of love because the man cannot conceptualize the woman as a person separate from her sexual and social need-fulfilling roles for him. Egregious narcissistic patterns victimize others, usually without violence.

What Heterosexuality Guarantees

Nothing much. Male heterosexuality per se guarantees nothing beyond a mental representation of females as sometimes sexually and romantically alluring. It is functionally characterized by a reflex arousal to the visualization or touch of the female body. When it works well, it is because the man correctly recognizes that he is in a sexual context; his reflex arousal mechanisms enable him to have sex with a partner. Because heterosexual men's construal of social contexts as sexual ones is not invariably the same as their partners, they have to learn to communicate, understand, and negotiate. These are acquired or learned skills, not reflexes. Sex is rarely a simple matter.

Living out here with real women. Because default heterosexuality is a private matter, enhanced through fantasies, the demands of development force men to exist outside themselves in the external world with real women. Default heterosexuality does not provide much reassurance to a woman about a man's capacity to love, abide, and be a sexually satisfying partner. Being heterosexually healthy means being able to exist in a real interpersonal sexual world. Being heterosexually limited often means living primarily in one's internal erotic world.

The impressive power of the default capacities. There is an inevitable tension between the demands of being a civilized heterosexual and the default appreciation of the sexual potentials of attractive women. The celebration of young women's beauty, however, remains at a visual and imaginary level in each man. This is endlessly reinforced by culture's celebration of these women. Men imagine that being the sexual partner of such a beauty would be marvelous. Their past personal experience with real women does not seem to have much power to modify their erotic imagination for many years. The determinants of sexual rapture are far greater than the typical heterosexual's rendering of it. Default heterosexuality, however, continues to exert a reality-distorting influence on the man's sensibilities, social judgments, and values. This is highly relevant to conceptualizing mental health. Prospective study of men's development has demonstrated a strong relationship between maturity, virtue, and psychological health (Vaillant 1993). More recently, prospective data analysis has demonstrated that the psychologically healthy have far better social and physical experiences throughout the life cycle (Vaillant 1998).

Intimacy Skills

Psychological intimacy is the transient occurrence in two people of some degree of solace, contentment, or excitement as the result of conversation and nonverbal communication. It is integral to the attainment of heterosexual developmental potentials and a fulfilling sexual life throughout the life cycle. The importance of psychological intimacy lies in the processes that it stimulates. Psychological intimacies are the basis of friendships and love relationships and are one of the best known enabling forces for sexual behaviors (Levine 1998b). Not every heterosexual man is capable of attaining and maintaining psychological intimacy with a partner. Those who cannot use intimacy become dependent on other stimuli (usually sources that derive from default heterosexuality—for example, images of women, sex with strangers, novelty seeking).

The First Step

Psychological intimacy begins with one person's ability to share his inner experiences with another. This capacity rests on three separate abilities of the speaker:

1. The capacity to know what one feels and thinks
2. The willingness to say it to another
3. The language skills to express the feelings and the ideas with words

Incapacity of any of these abilities limits the chance of establishing and maintaining psychological intimacy. For instance, some heterosexual men do not recognize what they feel, even when their feelings are intense. The best they can do is to say that they are "upset" before or after they behave in some problematic manner. Some men do not trust anyone enough to share their inner experiences. Others are limited by their language skills: they know what they are experiencing, but they cannot explain it. The crucial first step toward psychological intimacy is the sharing by one person of something from within the inner self. What is shared need not be elegantly said, lofty in its content, or unusual in any way. It just needs to be from the inner experience of the self—from the continual monologue of self-consciousness, from the speaker's subjectivity.

The Second Step

For intimacy to occur, the listener has to respond to the speaker in a manner that conveys:

- A noncritical acceptance of what is being said
- An awareness of the importance of the moment to the speaker
- A grasp of what is being said
- A pleasure in hearing what the speaker has to say

In ordinary social interactions, intimacy will not occur if a listener negatively judges what is being said (e.g., by saying, "You shouldn't feel that way.") or if the listener doesn't acknowledge the significance of what is being said (e.g., by remarking impatiently, "Can't this wait? Don't you see how busy I am?") or if the listener listens but misses the point of the speaker's words or misinterprets his partner's discussion as a request for a practical solution.

Why Is Intimate Conversation Pleasurable?

When two people perform their speaking and listening tasks reasonably well, they share a transient, rarefied pleasure. The pleasure has several components:

- The speaker's pleasure is in large part solace—a form of peace or contentment that results from sharing the inner self, being listened to with interest, and being comprehended. Solace is the response to being seen, known, understood, and accepted.
- The speaker experiences a sense of excitement and energy and an uplifting of mood.
- The speaker feels hope for a better future.
- The listener's pleasure and contentment result because the listener is trusted enough to be told, competent enough to

have enabled the telling, perceptive enough to accurately grasp the speaker's story, and wise enough to respond without censure.

Short-Term Consequences of New Psychological Intimacy

The reciprocal sharing of the inner monologue with a person who receives it well creates a bond between the speaker and the listener. Thereafter, each regards the other differently. They glance at each differently, touch each other differently, and laugh together differently and can continue to discuss readily other aspects of their private selves. These external manifestations are the result of a feeling of attachment, a loss of the usual social indifference, and an internal vision of the person as special. Intimate conversations ignite new processes. The listener and the speaker internalize one another. Internalization has predictable consequences, including the following:

- Imagining the person when she is not present
- Inventing conversations with her
- Preoccupation with her physical attributes
- Anticipation of the next opportunity to be together (i.e., missing the person)
- Dreaming about her
- Thinking about her as a sex partner

Weaving the Person Into the Psyche

When psychological intimacy occurs, we begin to weave the person into our selves. Our new intimate partner is not only reacted to as a unique individual, she stimulates thoughts, feelings, and worries that we previously experienced in relationship to others. When this process occurs in a psychotherapeutic intimacy, it is designated as transference. Transference, however, is the ordinary response to psychological intimacy.

Determinants of Eroticization

The speed of the eroticization provoked by intimacy is modified by at least seven factors: age, sex, sexual orientation, social status, purpose in talking together, nature of other emotional commitments, and the individuals' attitudes toward private sexual phenomena. If the pair consists of a comparably aged, socially eligible heterosexual man and woman, the eroticization triggered by sharing of some aspects of their inner selves can occur with lightning speed—in both of them. The stimulation of the erotic imagination may never occur, may take a long time to occur, or may occur only in a fleeting, disguised way, depending on how these seven factors line up.

Long-Term Consequences of Psychological Intimacy

Without repetition of the experience of solace and pleasure, the consequences of intimacy are short-lived. In order for psychological intimacy to bloom fully, periodic sharing of aspects of the inner self is required. There are good reasons to continue to share over time. Reattaining psychological intimacy provides a sense of security about the relationship. It calms the individuals. Intimacy allows people to be seen, known, accepted, understood, and treated with uniqueness. This is the stuff of being and staying in love and is the primary interpersonal stimuli to women's sexual desire. Heterosexual men may not like to admit it, but psychological intimacy is also the primary contextual stimulus for their desire. Most sexual partners expect to be dear friends. Lovers are expected to stabilize us. Psychological intimacy within a relationship creates personal stability, self-cohesion, self-esteem, and improved ego function (Frayn 1990).

Consequences of Losing Psychological Intimacy

When psychological intimacies disappear from previously important relationships, various anxiety, depressive, sexual, or somatic symptoms may appear or worsen. If healthy heterosexual development—being in love with a particular woman—requires intimacy skills, then abiding comfortably for a lifetime with that woman requires skills to maintain psychological intimacy even in the face of the unpredictable difficulties that occur during adulthood. Having once attained a high level of psychological intimacy, its loss is likely to place a person in a symptomatic, sad, and angry state. The loss of intimacy within a relationship is also a matter of shame and stigma for heterosexual men and may explain why it is so difficult for them to seek psychiatric care. Many men intuitively understand the implied heterosexual developmental potentials even if they do not think that these potentials are attainable in this modern era.

Women Are More Naturally Intimate

Compelling theories now exist about the essential psychological styles of girls and women and of boys and men (Gilligan 1982). In comparison with men, women typically require more frequent psychologically intimate experiences—with each other, with children, and with lovers or spouses. They complain more often about the lack of psychological intimacy in their relationships to men. Men are typically patterned to more autonomous operational patterns. They have trouble understanding why women complain about their lack of communicating, why they say their marriages do not contain enough intimacy. It is now more broadly recognized that psychologically healthy women organize their lives to a far greater degree around relationships—to friends, family, children, and lovers or spouses—than do healthy men. Women expect themselves to be relational, to gravitate to connection, and to personally evaluate their successes in terms of psychologically intimate relationships and responsiveness to other people's lives. Men tend to think of themselves as successful in terms of the creation of a unique, self-sufficient wage earner (Jordan 1989). These large generalizations about gender differences leave room for the fact that no one psychological trait is the exclusive province of either gender.

Psychological Intimacy Does Not Sustain Sexual Function for a Lifetime

Even heterosexual men who are capable of intimacy within a longstanding relationship find themselves mentally seeking sexual novelty or envying those who seem to have it. Couples who abide with each other well may be able to sustain sexual life longer than highly conflicted ones, but even they often find themselves searching for ways to enhance their sexual interest in one another. Psychological intimacy does not prevent individuals from aging, becoming physically ill, or being significantly affected by what happens in life outside of a marriage. Attaining the goals of heterosexual development does not prevent sex from losing its former luster; it does not immunize a man from boredom, discontent, envy, or fantasy. The heterosexual man's developmental line is often marked by private struggle between his sense of reality, his conscience, and his longings for a better existence for much of his life. These struggles seem to quiet down as the years add up.

References

Billy JOG, Tanfer K, Grady WR, et al: The sexual behavior of men in the United States. Fam Plann Perspect 25:52–60, 1993

Erickson EH: Childhood and Society, 2nd Edition. New York, WW Norton, 1963

Frayn DH: Intersubjective processes in psychotherapy. Can J Psychiatry 35:434–438, 1990

Freud S: Three essays on the theory of sexuality (1905), in the Standard Edition of the Complete Psychological Works of Sigmund Freud, Vol 7. Translated and edited by Strachey J. London, Hogarth Press, 1971, pp 135–243

Gilligan C: In a Different Voice: Psychological Theory and Women's Development. Cambridge, MA, Harvard University Press, 1982

Goldstein I, Padma-Nathan H, Rosen RC, et al: Sildenafil in the treatment of male erectile dysfunction. N Engl J Med 338:1397–1404, 1998

Green R: "Sissy Boy Syndrome" and the Development of Male Homosexuality. New Haven, CT, Yale University Press, 1987

Hines M, Collaer ML: Gonadal hormones and sexual differentiation of human behavior: developments from research on endocrine syndromes and studies of brain structure. Annual Review of Sex Research 4:1–48, 1993

Janssen E, Everaerd W: Determinants of male sexual arousal. Annual Review of Sex Research 4:211–246, 1993

Jordan JV: Relational development: therapeutic implications of empathy and shame. Work in Progress. Wellesley, MA, Stone Center Working Paper Series, 1989

Kafka MP: Hypersexual desire in males: an operational definition and clinical implications for males with paraphilias and paraphilia-related disorders. Arch Sex Behav 26:505–525, 1997

Kaplan HS: The Sexual Desire Disorders: Dysfunctional Regulation of Sexual Motivation. New York, Brunner/Mazel, 1995

Levine SB: Developing our sexual identity, in Sex Is Not Simple. Columbus, Ohio Psychology Publishing, 1988, pp 90–112

Levine SB: Erection problems, in Sexual Life: A Clinician's Guide. New York, Plenum, 1992, pp 120–142

Levine SB: The nature of love, in Sexuality in Mid-Life. New York, Plenum, 1998a, pp 1–23

Levine SB: Psychological intimacy, in Sexuality in Mid-Life. New York, Plenum, 1998b, pp 25–36

Levine SB: Some reflections on countertransference: a discussion of Dr. Derek Polonsky's presentation. Journal of Sex Education and Therapy 22:13–18, 1998c

Lewis JM: For better or worse: interpersonal relationships and individual outcome. Am J Psychiatry 155:582–589, 1998

Martinson FM: Childhood sexuality, in Handbook of Human Sexuality. Edited by Wolman BB, Money J (eds). Englewood Cliffs, NJ, Prentice-Hall, 1980, pp 29–59

McClintock MK, Herdt G: Rethinking puberty: the development of sexual attraction. Current Directions in Psychological Sciences 5:178–183, 1996

Melis M, Argiolas A, Gessa G: Apomorphine-induced penile erection and yawning: site of action in the brain. Brain Res 415:98–104, 1987

Montejo-Gonzalez AL, Llorca G, Izquierdo JA, et al: SSRI-induced sexual dysfunction: fluoxetine, paroxetine, sertraline, and fluvoxamine in a prospective, multicenter and descriptive study of 344 patients. J Sex Marital Ther 23:176–194, 1997

Nofzinger EA, Thase ME, Reynolds CF III, et al: Sexual function in depressed men: assessment by self-report, behavioral, and nocturnal penile tumescence measures before and after treatment with cognitive behavior therapy. Arch Gen Psychiatry 50:24–30, 1993

Pillard RC, Bailey JM: A biological perspective on sexual orientation. Psychiatr Clin North Am 18:71–84, 1995

Polonsky DC: What do you do when they won't do it? the therapeutic dilemma of low desire. Journal of Sex Education and Therapy 22:5–12, 1998

Rosen RC, Ashton AK: Prosexual drugs: empirical status of the "new aphrodisiacs." Arch Sex Behav 22:521–543, 1993

Rowland DL, Greenleaf WJ, Dorfman LJ, et al: Aging and sexual function in men. Arch Sex Behav 22:545–557, 1993

Sell RL: Defining and measuring sexual orientation: a review. Arch Sex Behav 26:643–658, 1997

Stoller RJ: The "bedrock" of masculinity and femininity: bisexuality. Arch Gen Psychiatry 26:207–212, 1972

Stoller RJ: Perversion: The Erotic Form of Hatred. New York, Pantheon, 1975

Vaillant G: The Wisdom of the Ego. Cambridge, MA, Harvard University Press, 1993

Vaillant G: Natural history of male psychological health; XIV: relationship of mood disorder vulnerability to physical health. Am J Psychiatry 155:184–191, 1998

Weinberg TS: Research in sadomasochism: a review of sociological and social psychological literature. Annual Review of Sex Research 5:257–279, 1994

Chapter 3

Evaluation and Treatment of Erectile Dysfunction

Stanley E. Althof, Ph.D., and Allen D. Seftel, M.D.

In March 1998, sildenafil citrate (Viagra) received approval by the Food and Drug Administration (FDA) for the treatment of erectile dysfunction. In the first 3 months, three million prescriptions were written, making it the most prescribed medication in the United States. Instantly the drug became a happening—with coverage on the front page of *The New York Times,* cartoons in *The New Yorker* magazine, jokes on *The Tonight Show* with Jay Leno and on *Late Show* with David Letterman, Internet sites offering to rush the drug to your door, former Senator Bob Dole stepping forward to acknowledge that, yes, he participated in the clinical trials, internists besieged by patients demanding the drug, legitimate and preposterous claims of the drug's efficacy, shocking stories of men dying while taking the drug, and researchers announcing to the media that the drug also enhanced the sexual lives of women.

Obviously, sildenafil transformed the treatment and research landscape. Its success eclipsed the scientific advances of the 1980s that elucidated the pathophysiology of erectile function and included the development of other innovative treatments for impotence. As these pre-sildenafil treatments (e.g., self-injections, vacuum devices, transurethral systems) became available—and because they were reversible, safe, and efficacious—the established principle of etiology guiding treatment became less meaningful. Before the introduction of these treatments, men diagnosed with psychogenic erectile dysfunction received treat-

Part of Dr. Seftel's work is supported by the Department of Veterans Affairs, VA Central Office, Washington, DC.

ment from mental health professionals, and those with organic dysfunction were seen by urologists or other health specialists. These therapies altered the traditional role of the mental health professional, which had been to 1) assess the etiology of erectile dysfunction, 2) offer psychotherapy to men or couples with primarily psychological dysfunction, or 3) treat the conspicuous psychological sequelae of organic conditions (Althof and Seftel 1995; Levine and Althof 1991). Once these treatments became available, the clinician's role was expanded to include identification and attenuation of resistances to medical treatments for erectile dysfunction.

This chapter seeks to update psychiatrists on the nosology, prevalence, and major risk factors regarding erectile dysfunction; review recent advances in understanding the physiology of erection; present a contemporary etiologic paradigm describing the interplay between psychological and biological variables; introduce a pragmatic cost-effective algorithm for evaluation and treatment of erectile problems; contrast the advantages and limitations of the current medical treatment options; and consider an expanded role for mental health clinicians.

Nosology: Impotence Versus Erectile Dysfunction

For years, the terms *impotence* and *erectile dysfunction* were used interchangeably to denote the inability of a man to achieve or maintain erection sufficient to permit satisfactory sexual intercourse (Krane et al. 1989). Social scientists objected to the impotence label, because of its pejorative implications and lack of precision (Rosen and Leiblum 1992). The National Institutes of Health (1992) advocated that the term erectile dysfunction be used in its place and defined it as the "inability of the male to achieve an erect penis as part of the overall multifaceted process of male sexual function." This definition de-emphasizes intercourse as the sine qua non of sexual life and gives equal importance to other aspects of male sexual behavior. Table 3–1 lists the DSM-IV diagnostic criterion set for male erectile disorder (American Psychiatric Association 1994).

Table 3–1. DSM-IV diagnostic criteria for male erectile disorder

A. Persistent or recurrent inability to attain, or to maintain until completion of the sexual activity, an adequate erection.
B. The disturbance causes marked distress or interpersonal difficulty.
C. The erectile dysfunction is not better accounted for by another Axis I disorder (other than a sexual dysfunction) and is not due exclusively to the direct physiological effects of a substance (e.g., a drug of abuse, a medication) or a general medical condition.

Specify type:

Lifelong type
Acquired type

Specify type:

Generalized type
Situational type

Specify:

Due to psychological factors
Due to combined factors

Source. Reprinted from American Psychiatric Association: *Diagnostic and Statistical Manual of Mental Disorders,* 4th Edition. Washington, DC, American Psychiatric Association, 1994. Used with permission.

DSM-IV asks the clinician to make three additional discriminations: 1) lifelong versus acquired, 2) generalized versus situational, and 3) due to psychological factors versus due to combined factors. When the dysfunction is due to medical factors or a substance, it is diagnosed as sexual dysfunction due to a general medical condition or as substance-induced sexual dysfunction.

Prevalence and Medical Risk Factors

At least 10–20 million American men experience erectile dysfunction. The most recent and comprehensive epidemiological report, the Massachusetts Male Aging Study (Feldman et al. 1994), asked men between the ages of 40 and 70 years to categorize their erectile function as completely, moderately, minimally, or not impotent. Fifty-two percent of the sample reported some dysfunction. This study demonstrated that erectile dysfunction is an age-dependent disorder: between the ages of 40 and 70 years the probability of complete impotence tripled from 5.1% to 15%, moderate impotence doubled from 17% to 34%, and minimal impotence remained constant at 17%. By age 70 years, only 32% of the sample population portrayed themselves as free of erectile dysfunction.

After the data were adjusted for age, men treated for diabetes (28%), heart disease (39%), and hypertension (15%) had significantly higher probabilities for erectile dysfunction than the sample as a whole (9.6%). Men with untreated ulcer (18%), arthritis (15%), and allergy (12%) were also significantly more likely to develop erectile dysfunction. Although erectile dysfunction was not associated with total serum cholesterol, the probability of dysfunction varied inversely with high-density lipoprotein cholesterol.

Certain classes of medication were related to increased probability for total erectile dysfunction. The percentage of men with complete dysfunction who were taking hypoglycemic agents (26%), antihypertensive drugs (14%), vasodilators (36%), and cardiac drugs (28%) was significantly higher than the sample as a whole (9.6%).

Finally, cigarette smoking increased the probability of total erectile dysfunction in men with treated heart disease, treated hypertension, or untreated arthritis. It similarly increased the probability for men on cardiac, antihypertensive, or vasodilator medications.

Various psychotropic medications, including antipsychotic medications, tricyclic antidepressants, and selective serotonin reuptake inhibitors, have been shown to cause erectile dysfunction (Aizenberg et al. 1995; Segraves 1998).

Physiology of Erection

Anatomy

The penis contains two paired corpora cavernosa and a corpus spongiosum. The corpus spongiosum surrounds the urethra and continues distally to form the glans penis. Each corpus cavernosum is surrounded by a thick fibrous sheath, the tunica albuginea, which encases the sponge-like cavernosal tissue with multiple interconnected sinusoidal, or lacunar, spaces lined by vascular endothelium. Interconnections between the corpus cavernosum and the corpus spongiosum allow blood to pass between the two chambers (Vardi et al. 1997). The walls of the lacunar spaces are composed of thick bundles of smooth muscle (the trabecular smooth muscle) and a fibroelastic frame that consists of fibroblasts, collagen, and elastin (Krane et al. 1989). The tunica is composed entirely of collagen.

The right and left cavernosal arteries, which are 600–1000 μm in diameter, are terminal branches of the hypogastric-pudendal arterial bed. Multiple muscular, corkscrew-shaped arteries (the helicine arteries), which are approximately 150 μm in size, branch off each cavernosal artery and open directly into the lacunar spaces. When constricted, these muscular vessels create a large pressure gradient between the cavernosal artery and the lacunar spaces (Kifor et al. 1997; Krane et al. 1989).

Neurovascular Factors

Erection is a neurovascular phenomenon. In the flaccid state the penis is under venous oxygen tension and pressure. During erection it is transformed into an arterial organ (Kim et al. 1993). This means that the penis in the flaccid state is akin to a large vein. It is characterized by venous blood pressure and venous oxygen tension. When erect, it becomes an arterial organ. The oxygen tension is now arterial, and the internal pressure should equal that of mean arterial pressure. Three neuroeffector systems control trabecular smooth muscle tone; they may also influence the penile blood vessel smooth muscle tone. Adrenergic nerves, endothelin, and angiotensin constrict penile blood vessel and corporal smooth muscle via norepinephrine or similar adrenergic agonists acting on α_1 adrenoceptors or on specific endothelin receptors (Gondre and Christ 1998; Saenz de Tejada et al. 1989). Endothelin is a family of peptides with potent vasoconstrictor effects. There are several molecules, such as endothelin-1 and endothelin-2 (ET-1, ET-2), that are 21 amino acids in length. Originally identified in endothelial cells, endothelin is now known to be present in many tissues (Peroutka 1994). Non-adrenergic-noncholinergic (NANC) nerves control initial blood vessel and corporal smooth muscle relaxation through the release of nitric oxide (NO), which facilitates relaxation via cyclic guanosine monophosphate (cGMP) formation (Azadzoi et al. 1992; Kim et al. 1991; Rajfer et al. 1992; Seftel et al. 1996; Simonsen et al. 1997) and changes in potassium conductance (Seftel et al. 1996). NANC nerves are autonomic nerves that travel along with cholinergic and other nerves through the pelvic plexus to innervate the penis. Researchers believe that NANC nerves do not contain acetylcholine, adrenaline, or noradrenaline. Thus they are noncholinergic (no acetylcholine for neurotransmission) and nonadrenergic (no noradrenaline or adrenaline for neurotransmission). Other minor vasodilatory systems include vasodilatory peptides such as cyclic adenosine monophosphate and vasoactive intestinal polypeptide. Cholinergic nerves appear to have a modulatory role over adrenergic and NANC nerves but do not exert a direct effect on the trabecular smooth muscle (Saenz de Tejada et al. 1988).

Nitric oxide mediates vasodilation of the penile vascular resistance bed and the cavernosal smooth muscle (Azadzoi et al. 1992; Burnett et al. 1992; Kim et al. 1991, 1993; Rajfer et al. 1992; Simonsen et al. 1997). NO synthesis is related to the increase from venous to arterial oxygen tension in the penis during erection (Kim et al. 1993). Vasodilation of the cavernosal and helicine arteries permits an increase in blood flow and pressure throughout the internal pudendal arterial system. Simultaneously, the trabecular smooth muscle that surrounds the lacunar spaces vasodilates (Krane et al. 1989; Lue and Tanagho 1987), allowing blood to enter the lacunar spaces. The systemic blood pressure, now transmitted through the dilated helicine arteries, expands the relaxed trabecular walls against the tunica albuginea. This compresses the plexus of subtunical venules, reduces lacunar space venous outflow, and elevates lacunar space pressure, making the penis rigid (Krane et al. 1989; Lue and Tanagho 1987). The pressure in the lacunar space during an erection is the result of the equilibrium between the perfusion pressure in the cavernosal and helicine arteries and the resistance to blood outflow through the compressed subtunical venules. The reduction of venous outflow by the mechanical compression of subtunical venules is known as the corporal veno-occlusive mechanism (Azadzoi et al. 1988; Lue and Tanagho 1987).

Detumescence is not well understood, but most likely, adrenergic stimulation induces vasoconstriction, decreasing the blood flow into and increasing the blood flow out of the penis, returning the penis to the flaccid state.

Molecular Evidence of Nitric Oxide Production

The production of NO is mediated by a family of nitric oxide synthase (NOS) enzymes that represent distinct gene products. These enzymes produce NO through a complex set of reduction-oxidation reactions that result in the conversion of L-arginine to L-citrulline (Bush et al. 1992). The isoforms of NOS have been categorized as being either inducible (induced to form in response to certain agonists such as bacterial toxins) or constitutive (present at all times, part of the normal physiologic milieu). The inducible isoform of NOS (iNOS) is associated primarily with macrophages and is activated by specific cytokines as part of the immune response. The endothelial and neuronal isoforms of NOS (eNOS and nNOS, respectively) are constitutive and activated in part by an increased concentration of intracellular calcium and calmodulin binding to the enzyme (Burnett et al. 1992).

Experimental evidence suggests that the constitutive isoforms of NOS may be responsible for NO production in penile erection. Recent evidence suggests that eNOS and its subsequent production of NO may be a significant route of NO-mediated cavernosal relaxation. For example, transgenic mice lacking nNOS are still capable of erectile activity with pelvic nerve stimulation (Burnett et al. 1996).

The eNOS, nNOS, and iNOS isoforms of nitric oxide synthase in the human penis have recently been identified (Burnett et al. 1992; Seftel et al. 1997). Identification of the molecular mechanisms of erectile dysfunction will allow broader therapeutic strategies to be developed.

Gap Junctions

The penis is composed of a coordinated signaling network that enables the cascading sequence to culminate in erection. Researchers discovered that penile corporal tissue relaxation and contraction are coordinated events governed by intracellular communications known as *gap junctions* (Christ et al. 1993). This allows rapid corporal smooth muscle cell-to-cell communication through a milieu of smooth muscle fibers, extracellular matrix, and collagen.

Pathophysiology of Erectile Dysfunction: Aging and Diabetes-Related Disease

A new area of investigation into age- and diabetes-related impotence concerns the role of penile advanced glycation products. The extracellular matrix undergoes progressive changes during senescence that are characterized by decreased solubility, decreased digestibility, increased heat denaturation time, and accumulation of yellow and fluorescent material (Sell and Monnier 1989). These changes, such as tissue stiffening, affect particularly collagen rich tissues, such as tendons and arteries, and are thought to result from the formation of age-related protein-sugar cross-links mediated by the advanced glycation (Maillard) reaction. Elucidation of the structure of these cross-links, known as advanced glycation end-products (AGEs), has been of major interest to gerontologists and collagen chemists for two reasons. First, an inverse relationship exists between mammalian longevity and the aging rate of collagen, suggesting that the process that governs longevity may express itself in the aging rate of collagen. Second, the progressive increase in stiffness of collagen-rich tissues (e.g., arteries, lungs, joints, extracellular matrix) has been associated with age-related diseases such as hypertension, emphysema, decreased joint mobility, and inability to fight infections.

These cross-links were shown to contain a pentose-mediated

protein named pentosidine (Monnier et al. 1984). In patients with diabetes and chronic renal failure, pentosidine levels increase with aging in plasma, skin, and other tissues. Plasma pentosidine levels tend to return toward normal with hemodialysis or renal transplantation (Hricik et al. 1993). Accelerated increases in penile pentosidine and pyrroline deposition were found in both the tunica albuginea and the corpus cavernosum in impotent diabetic males (Seftel et al. 1997). A time-dependent accumulation of AGEs in the aging penis might similarly attenuate the NO required for penile corporal smooth muscle relaxation. With aging cavernosal relaxation may be attenuated because of altered posttranslational eNOS activity and a decreased intracellular calcium level (Haas et al. 1998). From these pathophysiologic studies new therapeutic strategies will be developed based on the molecular understanding of erectile dysfunction.

Hypoxemia

Hypoxemia could be a cause of erectile dysfunction. Penile NO synthesis appears to depend on the change from a venous to an arterial oxygen tension. A lack of full arterial oxygen tension might attenuate penile NO synthesis and the resultant vasodilation required for erection.

Moreland and colleagues (Nehra et al. 1996) postulated that chronic hypoxemia produces an upregulation of transforming growth factor β (TGFβ), which induces corpus cavernosal fibrosis. Indeed, the cavernosal tissue, which has a 40%–45% smooth muscle content, shifts to an increase in collagen deposition at the expense of the smooth muscle, which now is reduced to 30%–35% of the total content. By examining cavernosal smooth muscle, Seftel (1999) concluded that male erectile dysfunction is an active process characterized by a loss of apoptosis. His data support the concept of hypoxemia-mediated erectile dysfunction via upregulation of P53 but do not substantiate a role for TGFβ in male erectile dysfunction.

Researchers have identified two distinct sources for the hypoxemia: pulmonary, based on hypoventilation and pulmonary microembolization; and anemia, based on diminished erythropoietin production (De Broe and De Backer 1989; Eckardt and Kurtz 1989). Hypoxemia also increases the release of local constricting factors such as endothelin, resulting in further increases in smooth muscle vascular tone (Simonson et al. 1992). Recent studies have shown that treatment of the anemia of chronic renal failure with recombinant human erythropoietin improves systemic hemodynamics, including increased cardiac output, decreased peripheral resistance, increased tissue oxygenation, and improved sexual function (De Broe and De Backer 1989; Nonnast-Daniel et al. 1988). Increases in tissue oxygenation could positively influence the erectile mechanism by promoting NO release and sustaining corporal smooth muscle relaxation.

Gene Therapy

Gene therapy is a new and exciting area of research and treatment. It involves replacing the abnormal or defective gene responsible for impotence with a new copy of the gene. Currently two strategies address this issue. Garban et al. (1997) attempted to place iNOS into the rat penis to allow for increased NO production, whereas Christ et al. (1998) sought to alter the potassium channels of DNA in a rat model. Christ et al. (1998) demonstrated that the intracorporal microinjection of pCMVβ/ Lac Z DNA in 10-week-old rats resulted in significant incorporation and expression of β-galactosidase activity in 10 of 12 injected animals for up to 75 days postinjection. Moreover, electrical stimulation of the cavernous nerve revealed that, relative to the responses obtained in age-matched control animals ($N = 12$), intracavernous injection of naked pcDNA/hSlo DNA was associated with a statistically significant elevation in the mean amplitude of the intracavernous pressure response at all levels of current stimulation (range 0.5–10 mA) at both 1 month ($N = 5$) and 2 months ($N = 8$) postinjection. Qualitatively similar observations were made at 3 and 4 months postinjection. These data indicate that naked hSlo DNA is quite easily incorporated into corporal smooth muscle and that expression is sustained for at least 2 months in corporal smooth muscle cells in vivo. Finally, after expression, hSlo is capable of measurably altering nerve-stimulated penile erection. These data provide compelling evidence for the potential utility of gene therapy in the treatment of erectile dysfunction.

Integration of Biological and Psychiatric Theories: The Interactive Etiologic Model Paradigm

Prior to 1980 erectile dysfunction was conceptualized in binary terms: it was either psychogenic or organic. When fewer treatment options were available, this paradigm simplified treatment planning. Patients with psychogenic erectile dysfunction were referred for psychotherapy, patients deficient in testosterone received hormone replacement, and patients with other organic conditions were referred for penile prostheses.

The development of oral medications; self-injection, vacuum tumescence therapy, and transurethral therapies; and vascular surgery complicated the decision tree. Clinicians recognized that many patients failed to fit neatly into either a psychogenic or an organic category. A third category, mixed erectile disorder, evolved to account for those patients with both psychological and organic factors, yet the notion of "mixed" conveys a static rather than dynamic interactive concept.

This tripartite model gave way to an interactive paradigm in which psychological and medical factors are conceptualized as dynamically additive (Levine 1992; LoPiccolo 1992; Schnarf 1990; Tiefer and Melman 1989). This model captures the ever-changing influences of biology and psychological life. Regardless of the precipitating causes, changes occur over time in both domains. This model encompasses 1) the psychological impact that the dysfunction has on the man and on the couple's sexual equilibrium, and 2) the fluctuating influence of medication, lifestyle, and disease.

This interactive model enables stepwise treatment recommendations in the psychological and biological domains. For instance, a couple might first be referred for time-limited psychological counseling to help pave the way for a future medical intervention. The model also explains the failure of treatments for biological problems that ignore psychological contributions.

Process of Care Model

Developed by a multidisciplinary panel of experts in family medicine, internal medicine, endocrinology, psychiatry, psychology, and urology, the process of care (POC) model guides clinicians in the diagnosis and treatment of erectile dysfunction (Rosen et al. 1998). Four guiding principles direct this model:

1. Identification and recognition of erectile dysfunction and its associated concomitant medical and psychological factors
2. A goal-directed, stepwise (with regard to the degree of invasiveness of diagnostic and treatment procedures and the degree of involvement of nonmedical specialists) treatment process for addressing patient and partner needs and preferences
3. Patient and partner education and communication
4. Clear guidelines for follow-up and referral

Six phases constitute the POC model. We discuss these phases in detail in the sections that follow.

Phase I

In the first phase, the clinician concentrates on establishing a primary diagnosis of erectile dysfunction. This is important because many patients incorrectly label problems with desire and ejaculation as "impotence" because of a lack of sophistication regarding normal sexual function. This phase is best accomplished through collaborative efforts on the part of the urologist and the mental health professional. In addition to conducting a physical examination and ordering appropriate laboratory studies, both professionals gather information about the man's past and present sexual function, illness, medication, lifestyle (e.g., smoking, drinking, diet), concomitant psychiatric problems (e.g., depression, anxiety, situational disturbance), the couple's relationship, and the social framework in which their lives are embedded.

Patient Assessment

The clinician outlines the history of the dysfunction and asks the patient to rate the current quality of erections on a 10-point scale (with 10 being the best erection) under a variety of circumstances: upon awakening, with fantasy, during masturbation, during foreplay, during intercourse, and with another partner. The clinician also elicits unusual or disturbing life circumstances coincident with the dysfunction.

The clinician examines other relevant parameters of sexual life, including sexual drive, frequency of lovemaking, orgasmic difficulties, and sexual satisfaction. Sometimes it is important to inquire about gender identity and paraphilia, as conflicts in these realms may produce erectile dysfunction.

The clinician assesses the magnitude of performance anxiety (Masters and Johnson 1970) and the forces that disrupt arousal. Dysfunction typically heightens concerns about masculinity. For example, the patient may think, "My penis is too small," or "A real man's penis gets hard anywhere, anytime, and under any circumstances." The clinician examines the quality of the couple's nonsexual relationship and conflicts emanating from other sources (e.g., work, finances, partner's health, difficulties with parents or children). It is important to evaluate the patient's motivation for resuming coitus and past utilization of specific treatment options. At this point the clinician ascertains obstacles to effective utilization of treatment alternatives (psychotherapeutic or medical).

Because erectile dysfunction affects the patient, his partner, and their nonsexual relationship, any evaluation that does not include the partner risks missing vital psychological information. Not infrequently the partner offers the clinician factual information that the patient omitted, for example, "Did he tell you about . . . his drinking problem, not getting a promotion, his affair, our daughter's drug problem, his mother's death, my mastectomy?" The clinician can assess possible partner sexual dysfunction and identify attitudes that are antithetical to resuming sexual life. The clinician may also reassure the partner by dispelling groundless self-recriminations and faulty self-attributions.

Clinicians will encounter resistance from some patients when they are asked to bring in their partners. For example, a patient might respond, "It's my problem, not hers" or "I don't want to embarrass her." Some of these protests yield to brief explanations. To collude with these resistances reinforces the destructive notion that the patient is the source of the problem; nonetheless, some patients refuse to invite their partners.

Urologic History and Physical Examination

The urologic history and physical examination focus on contributing organic factors. The urologic history notes the progression, consistency, and duration of the erectile dysfunction and raises questions concerning orgasm and libido.

Through the history, the clinician aims to identify underlying vascular risk factors such as hypertension, hyperlipidemia, cigarette smoking, diabetes mellitus, coronary heart disease, and peripheral vascular disease. The history includes questions about prior aortoiliac surgery, perineal or pelvic trauma, or pelvic radiation. A neurogenic etiology is suggested by neurologic disease (e.g., multiple sclerosis, spinal cord injury), pelvic surgery (e.g., radical cystoprostatectomy, proctocolectomy), or changes in bladder and bowel function or penile sensation and disorders associated with peripheral neuropathy (e.g., alcoholism, diabetes mellitus). Because of the association between certain drugs and erectile dysfunction, the clinician should obtain a detailed history of the patient's medications.

Physical examination includes evaluation of endocrine, neurologic, and vascular systems and local penile factors. Normal secondary sex characteristics such as body and facial hair patterns and normal external genitalia provide a gross index of androgen stimulation. Neurologic examination focuses on sacral dermatomes and includes sensory testing of the penis and perineum and evaluation of the bulbocavernosus reflex. The vascular examination involves the assessment of the arteries in the penis and lower extremities. The physician retracts the foreskin, examines the glans penis, evaluates the urethral meatus, and examines the penis for plaques or other dermatologic conditions. Penile plaques can be associated with Peyronie's disease. The physician palpates the entire corpus spongiosum for scarring, which can indicate urethral stricture disease or other urethral pathology, and examines the scrotum and testicles for dermatologic abnormalities, hernia, hydrocele, epididymitis, varicocele, and testicular tumors. Through the rectal examination the physician evaluates the bulbocavernosus reflex, prostatic size and shape, and anal pathology.

Laboratory tests are used to screen for low serum testosterone and high prolactin levels. In patients who are not regularly followed by an internist, additional tests for diabetes mellitus and hyperlipidemia are useful.

Phase II

The second phase begins with the clinician reviewing the initial findings, discussing referral if indicated, and beginning an educational process. Education entails an in-depth discussion of all the treatment options with the benefits and limitations of each. Material prepared by the clinician, supplemented with pharmaceutical pamphlets, videos, or hands-on demonstration is often helpful in educating the couple. By fostering the patient's or couple's awareness, reviewing expectations from treatment, and correcting unrealistic desires, the clinician promotes an attitude that the patient and doctor are on the same side. Such an approach is likely to engender enhanced patient compliance.

At this point additional diagnostic testing is often indicated to further clarify etiology, to gratify the patient's wish to know what is causing the dysfunction, or for medico-legal reasons. Frequently used tests include nocturnal penile tumescence testing, dynamic infusion cavernosometry/cavernosography, and duplex ultrasonography.

Phase III

The third phase focuses on modifying reversible causes of the erectile dysfunction. Among the reversible causes are offending prescription or nonprescription (including recreational) drugs; modifiable behaviors such as cigarette smoking, alcohol abuse, partner conflict, and lifestyle patterns that diminish intimacy (e.g., workaholism); specific endocrinologic conditions; and pelvic trauma or anatomic defect. Sometimes simple medication or lifestyle alterations are sufficient to reverse the dysfunction.

Phase IV

Oral erectogenic agents, vacuum tumescence therapy, and couples or sexual counseling are considered first-line treatments for erectile dysfunction, based on their efficacy, reversibility, and modest side effect profile.

Oral Agents

Sildenafil acts by inhibiting the enzyme that breaks down cGMP. The enzyme that cleaves the cGMP monophosphate bond is known as type 5 phosphodiesterase and is found predominantly in the penis. Sildenafil is a type 5 phosphodiesterase inhibitor (Goldstein et al. 1998). Sildenafil enhances the man's ability to achieve a natural erection, given adequate psychic and physical stimulation. Unlike other interventions such as self-injection or transurethral or vacuum therapies, sildenafil does not induce erection irrespective of the man's degree of arousal. Although myths abound, sildenafil does not improve libido, prolong erection, promote spontaneous erections, or increase the size of the penis.

Sildenafil, taken on an empty stomach, works in approximately 1 hour. The only contraindications to sildenafil are the concomitant use of nitrate medications and the diagnosis of retinitis pigmentosa. Patients taking any form of nitrovasodilator can experience serious and significant drops in blood pressure, nearly 40 mm Hg systolic and 20 mm Hg diastolic (data on file, Pfizer Inc.), which may have serious cardiac consequences. Recreational use of amyl nitrite is also likely to produce the same significant drop in blood pressure. Sildenafil has no interaction with other medications, including antihypertensives, blood thinners, antidepressants, and drugs used to treat diabetes. Indeed, sildenafil works well in men who have hypertension, including those currently taking medications for their disease. It also helps men who have type 1 or type 2 diabetes, spinal cord injury, post–radical prostatectomy, or depression. Depending on the etiology of the dysfunction, sildenafil efficacy is 40%–70%. Table 3–2 lists the most common side effects associated with sildenafil use.

Data have been gathered on the long-term (i.e., 1 year) use of sildenafil in over 2,000 men (data on file, Pfizer Inc.). The drug comes in 25-, 50-, or 100-mg doses, and over 60% of men use the 100-mg dose. The long-term side effects parallel the short-term side effects. Sildenafil appears to be safe and effective over the course of at least 1 year. Recently published results of the early sildenafil trial describe the aforementioned experience (Goldstein et al. 1998).

Several other agents are under phase 1, 2, or 3 study. Apomorphine (TAP) works centrally on the medial preoptic area to produce an erection. Early data suggest a significant improvement in erectile activity over placebo. The main side effect appears to be nausea, which is counteracted with an oral antiemetic. Other oral agents include Vasomax and a yet unnamed type 5 phosphodiesterase inhibitor in development by the ICOS Corporation. The data are insufficient at present to reach conclusions about these agents.

Yohimbine, a natural herb derived from the bark of an African

Table 3–2. Side effects of sildenafil therapy

Side effect	Incidence (%)	Cause
Headache and facial flushing	10	Vasodilatory effects of sildenafil on the cerebral circulation
Dyspepsia	5	Small overlap in sildenafil activity with type 4 phosphodiesterase found at the gastroesophageal sphincter, leaving the gastroesophageal sphincter open
Red-blue color vision changes or blurry vision	3	Slight overlap with type 6 phosphodiesterase, which exists in the retina

tree, has been used anecdotally for years in men with various forms of erectile dysfunction. Few objective, placebo-controlled studies validate the use of yohimbine. It is often given to patients who insist on an oral agent or as a placebo.

Vacuum Tumescence Therapy

Vacuum devices consist of several components: a clear plastic cylinder, a hand pump, lubricant, and tension rings. Battery-operated systems are available for men who are unable to pump the device manually. To create an erection the man places the clear plastic tube over his lubricated penis. Pumping creates an erection by producing a negative-pressure "vacuum" to draw blood into the corpora. The tension band is positioned on the base of the penis to maintain the erection. Active physiologic mechanisms underlie self-injection, whereas passive mechanisms are responsible for vacuum tumescence therapy (Diedrichs et al. 1989).

Ninety percent of men were able to achieve erections sufficient for intercourse by using this treatment alternative (Cooper 1987; Koreman et al. 1990; Nadig 1989; Nadig et al. 1986; Turner et al. 1990; Witherington 1989). Dropout rates are approximately 20% (Turner et al. 1991).

The common side effects associated with vacuum tumescence therapy are hematomas, ecchymosis, and petechiae; pain; numbness of the penis; pulling of scrotal tissue into the cylinder; and blocked and painful ejaculation (Althof and Turner 1992). Blood dyscrasias, penile bends, and anticoagulant therapy are relative contraindications.

Psychotherapy or Sexual Counseling

Psychotherapy aims to restore the man's potency to the optimal level possible, given the limits of physical well-being and life circumstances. The goal is to surmount the psychological and relational barriers that preclude mutual sexual satisfaction. The therapist attempts to transform the psychosomatic symptom of impotence into a cognitive and emotional experience. Psychodynamically oriented therapists view the dysfunction as a metaphor in which the man or couple are trying to simultaneously conceal and express conflictual aspects of themselves or the relationship. In symbolic terms the dysfunction contains a compromised solution to one of life's dilemmas (Althof 1989). Alternatively, behavior therapists understand the dysfunction as a maladaptive response to interpersonal or environmental occurrences.

The current psychotherapeutic approach to erectile dysfunction is an integration of psychodynamic, systems, behavioral, and cognitive approaches within a short-term psychotherapy model. An emphasis is placed on the sexual equilibrium and context. The guiding principles of treatment are to clarify the meaning of the symptom and understand the context in which it occurs or to learn alternative and more adaptive responses to stimulus.

For a small minority of couples, permission to be sexual may be all that is necessary (Annon 1974). Others may benefit from some education but most require more intensive treatment. Individual treatment is generally recommended for men with primary, or lifelong, erectile dysfunction. In these instances the symptom tends to mirror an intrapsychic developmental failure rather than an interpersonal conflict. In contrast, couple's treatment is customarily prescribed when the dysfunction is secondary, or acquired. In these situations, the symptom may represent the couple's shared solution to some aspect of their relationship or an adaptation to a recent crisis.

Psychotherapy improves sexual function in the man or couple by helping them to 1) express and accept difficult feelings regarding onerous life circumstances, 2) find new solutions for old problems, 3) surmount barriers to intimacy, 4) increase communication, 5) lessen performance anxiety, 6) transform destructive attitudes that interfere with lovemaking, and 7) modify rigid sexual repertoires. Patients come to understand how the dysfunction serves as their friend by protecting them from confronting unpleasant dilemmas (Althof 1989).

Psychotherapy also helps to reconstruct the commonly held mechanistic perspective regarding arousal (Zilbergeld 1992). Simply stated, men believe that the penis should become erect under any circumstance. The therapist enlightens the couple that how they feel about each other, the circumstances of their lives, and the conditions under which they make love influence their arousal.

Several excellent books, chapters, and articles devoted to the psychotherapy of erectile dysfunction are available (e.g., Althof 1989; Levine 1992; Levine and Althof 1991; Rosen et al. 1994). These explicate psychotherapeutic technique in detail.

Men with lifelong and acquired erectile dysfunctions usually achieve significant gains both initially and over the long term following participation in sex therapy. Men with acquired disorders tend to fare better than those with lifelong problems. Masters and Johnson (1970) reported initial failure rates of 41% for primary impotence and 26% for secondary impotence. Five years later these failure rates were 41% and 31% for primary and secondary dysfunctions, respectively. Several other well-controlled investigations (e.g., DeAmicus et al. 1985; Hawton et al. 1992; Heiman and LoPiccolo 1983; Kilmann et al. 1987; Reynolds 1991) have demonstrated the efficacy of psychological interventions for erectile dysfunctions, although none of these studies has achieved the impressive results of Masters and Johnson's original study.

In an excellent review of studies of erectile dysfunction, Mohr and Beutler (1990, p. 134) write that the "component parts of these treatments typically include behavioral, cognitive, systemic and interpersonal communications interventions. . . . Averaging across studies, it appears that approximately two-thirds of the men suffering from erectile failure will be satisfied with their improvement at follow-up ranging from six weeks to six years."

All studies with long-term follow-up noted a tendency for men to experience relapses. Hawton and Catalan (1986) reported that 75% of couples experienced "recurrence of, or continuing difficulty with, the presenting sexual problem"; this caused little to no concern for 34%. Patients indicated that they discussed the difficulty with the partner, practiced the techniques learned during therapy, accepted that difficulties were likely to recur and read books about sexuality. These techniques were effective coping strategies, in contrast to couples who stopped having sex or pretended that nothing was wrong. Hawton et al. (1992) suggest that positive treatment outcome is associated with better pretreatment communication and general sexual adjustment, especially the female partner's interest in and enjoyment of sex, absence of a psychiatric history in the woman, and the couple's willingness to complete homework.

Phase V

At the fifth phase, second-line treatments consisting of self-injection and transurethral therapy are considered for men or couples who decline or do poorly with first-line treatments.

Intracavernosal Self-Injection Therapy

As its name implies, self-injection is the introduction of a vasoactive compound via injection to the corporal bodies of the penis. The three medications most widely used to induce erection are papaverine hydrochloride, phentolamine (Regitine), and prostaglandin E_1 (Edex or Caverjet). Only prostaglandin E_1 has received FDA approval for treatment of erectile dysfunction (Linet and Ogrinc 1996), and it is the drug used most frequently by the majority of clinicians to treat erectile dysfunction. Papaverine and phentolamine are secondarily used to treat erectile dysfunction but have never received approval for this indication. Often the three medications are mixed in a compound known as trimix. The dose is titrated to produce an erection that lasts 30–60 minutes. Injections are given at the base of the penis at the 3 or 9 o'clock positions (posterolateral, away from the neurovascular bundle and urethra) using a disposable 1-ml insulin syringe and 26- to 30-gauge needle.

Self-injection therapy is most effective for patients with neurogenic problems, such as those with spinal cord injuries (Bodner et al. 1987; Sidi et al. 1987). It is least effective in men who have severe corporal veno-occlusive dysfunction or arterial insufficiency (Krane et al. 1989). Although not the principal option for treatment of erectile dysfunction with psychogenic etiologies, it may serve as an adjunct therapy to psychological intervention (Turner et al. 1989).

Based on the combined results of several studies, self-injection therapy was efficacious in 79%–91% of cases (Althof et al. 1991;

Virag et al. 1991). Although efficacious, approximately 50% of men who are referred for or who begin treatment drop out (Althof et al. 1989; Sidi et al. 1988).

Table 3–3 lists the major side effects of self-injection therapy (Althof and Turner 1992; Brown et al. 1998; Levine et al. 1989; Zentgraf et al. 1989). There are excellent long-term follow-up data demonstrating the relative safety and efficacy of intracavernosal injections.

Transurethral Therapy

Transurethral therapy came into being through the development of an innovative drug delivery system that allowed medication to be applied directly to the urethral mucosa. The major advantage of this treatment method is that it obviates the need to inject the penis to create an erection. Medication placed onto the urethral mucosa is transferred through vascular channels to the corpora cavernosum resulting in erection (Vardi and Saenz de Tejada 1997). The Vivus Corporation developed the medicated urethral system for erection (MUSE), which deposits a semisolid pellet of prostaglandin E_1 directly onto the urethral mucosa. This proprietary drug delivery system consists of a polypropylene applicator with a hollow stem 3.2 cm long and 3.5 mm in diameter. Prostaglandin E_1 in one of four predetermined dose levels (125, 250, 500, or 1,000 kg) is contained within the tip of the applicator.

Prior to using MUSE, patients are instructed to void so that residual urine provides a natural lubricant for the slow and gentle insertion of the stem into the urethra. A button on the crown of the applicator is depressed, depositing the pellet approximately 3 cm into the urethra. The applicator is then withdrawn. An erectile response is evident within 10 minutes that lasts 30–60 minutes.

In double-blind, placebo-controlled studies, Padma-Nathan et al. (1997) and Williams et al. (1998) reported that 43% of patients using MUSE had intercourse on at least one occasion. Lewis (1998) reported that by using an external constriction device, the Actis ring, approximately 60% of patients were able to achieve intercourse. MUSE is effective in producing a grade 3–4 erection in men who had spinal cord injuries with residual upper motor

Table 3–3. Side effects of self-injection therapy

Side effect	Frequency
Prolonged erection (priapism)	Occurs only occasionally as most patients are well instructed and properly titrated prior to initiation of therapy at home. It occurs less frequently when prostaglandin E_1 is the sole intracavernosal agent. Priapism occurs more commonly with papaverine or with trimix.
Fibrotic nodules with or without subsequent penile curvature	Common after 1 year
Liver function abnormalities	Rare and clinically insignificant
Bruising	Frequent but usually insignificant
Vasovagal episodes	Rare
Pain	Common
Infection	Unknown

neuronal function, but Bodner et al. (1987) found that erection created by MUSE was less acceptable to the 15 patients tested than the erection created by intracavernosal self-injection therapy.

Table 3–4 lists the most common side effects of transurethral therapy. Vaginal burning or itching was noted by 5.8% of female partners, and a condom barrier is recommended if the female partner is pregnant.

Phase VI

Only one intervention, implantation of a penile prosthesis, is designated as a third-line treatment. The penile prosthesis is a time-honored method of treating erectile dysfunction. Two types exist: a malleable or semirigid prosthesis and a multicomponent, inflatable penile prosthesis. The more components that make up

Table 3–4. Side effects of transurethral therapy

Side effect	Incidence (%)
Penile pain	32
Urethral burning	12
Minor urethral bleeding or spotting	5
Flu symptoms	4
Priapism and cavernosal fibrosis	less than 0.1

the device, the more that may go wrong with it. Complications include an infection rate of 1%–5%; possible urethral perforation during corporeal dilation, precluding device placement; and inadequate sizing, resulting in a cosmetic deformity. An experienced implanter will achieve success in 90%–95% of patients (Mulcahy 1997). The malleable prosthesis is relatively easy to insert. It is well suited for those patients with impaired manual dexterity and offers good concealment during daily activities.

The inflatable prosthesis requires an experienced surgeon for insertion. It gives a more natural erection as a result of its ability to inflate and deflate. Goldstein et al. (1998) recently demonstrated that the placement of the "Alpha1" three-piece inflatable prosthesis (Mentor Corporation) was successful in the majority of patients implanted. In a large multi-institutional study of 112 patients, Goldstein et al. (1998) reported a high degree of patient satisfaction. Complications included perioperative infection (2%), device malfunction (4%), and reoperation (9%).

New Roles for Mental Health Clinicians

First- and second-line treatments have dramatically changed the role of the mental health clinician. Because the medical interventions are safe, efficacious, and reversible, one could argue that patients with psychogenic dysfunction should first be considered for a medical intervention. Some prominent urologists have jokingly predicted that sex therapists should contemplate plans for early retirement (A. Melman, personal communication, August 1998).

We offer a more optimistic and contradictory set of ideas regarding the role of the mental health clinician. These notions are rooted in the two unexplained phenomena: 1) at least 85% of the population with erectile dysfunction do not avail themselves of treatment; and 2) although the medical treatments have impressive efficacy rates of 44%–91%, there is an equally impressive rate of discontinuation of 20%–50% (Althof and Turner 1992). This dropout rate is clearly not the result of a lack of efficacy or unwanted side effects; it appears to be a multiply determined response, motivated in part by psychological resistance to using a medical intervention and in part by interpersonal issues. Medical therapies address only the end organ; they cannot ameliorate the associated psychological and emotional concerns that obviate the efficacy of these treatments. Some urologists are too focused on producing an erection and bypass the emotional sequelae associated with erectile dysfunction. It is as if the physician is saying, "We can get it up. The rest is up to you." In the language of ego psychology, the mental health clinician's new role is to identify and attenuate resistance to treatment.

Here is what is typically seen: A 54-year-old married man with erectile dysfunction waits 2 years before seeking help. He felt puzzled, embarrassed, disgraced, weakened, and frightened, and during this time a pernicious pattern evolved. He began to go to sleep earlier or later than his partner or to offer plausible excuses for being too tired or too busy to make love. Aging also offered a convenient excuse. For example, he might say, "Look dear, I'm not 25 anymore." His goal was to avoid embarrassment or outright failure. The frequency of his attempts at lovemaking slowly dwindled to once a month, then once every several months, and then silently disappeared. He now has no desire and has become overly involved with work, television, volunteer efforts, or the children. He feels dysphoric, irritable, and defensive. Not only has intercourse disappeared but so has affectionate touch. He avoids anything that his partner might perceive remotely as a sexual invitation.

Over the same time period, his partner has begun to wonder, "Does he still love me?" "Is he having an affair?" "Is he not attracted to me anymore because of the weight I've gained over the years?" "Is that part of our relationship over?" Women often collude with their partners to avoid sexual activity, either to lessen their own pain of feeling rejected or to bring welcome relief from a previously unenjoyable activity. For many women, however, the relationship feels emptier with no lovemaking or affectionate touch.

After receiving treatment by the urologist, the patient may display his new medically engineered erection to his partner without discussion or prelude. Surprised because she was unaware of the patient's visit to the doctor, the partner may feel an amalgam of amazement, anger, dismay, and anxiety, for example, "Can I get ready for this again?" "Will this erection last?" "I was hoping we were past this." He, too, is anxious about his performance. Both feel awkward, embarrassed, and uncomfortable. Between them, the experience is less than memorable and somehow his desire to try again wanes. In reaction to this situation the patient may blame sildenafil, the vacuum device, MUSE, or injection therapy, saying they don't produce a "good-enough erection." A more careful inquiry often leads to the discovery that the formidable barriers of fear and anxiety that have been set in place by years of avoidance and failure were too difficult to surmount.

What the couple needs now is help overcoming these unseen intransigent blocks to much or all of their lovemaking. The mental health clinician is well suited to work with the couple (ideally) or with the man to illuminate and work through resistances to lovemaking that result from the painful period of abstinence and sometimes from ongoing relationship problems. The therapist can help the couple cultivate a romantic ambiance and engage in conversations that will physically and psychologically prepare them to become lovers again. The therapist can also assist them in accepting the changes that have occurred in their lives: menopause, disability, illness, or other life stresses. Sometimes these resistances need to be worked through prior to beginning a medical intervention. At other times they can be addressed simultaneously. If not confronted, these forces can render ineffectual the best-intentioned medical treatment efforts.

Powerful psychological resistances may be contributing to the high drop-out rates observed with the new mechanical and pharmaceutical treatments (data on sildenafil are not yet available). Not even sildenafil, as impressive as it seems, will prematurely end the careers of mental health professionals interested in treating sexual problems. Instead, these interventions will expand the traditional clinician role to identifying and helping patients or couples to overcome the resistances to effective utilization of medical treatments. By helping couples surmount these obstacles we can help them to enjoy once again the satisfaction of a loving sexual relationship.

The Future

No doubt other oral agents will be introduced to compete with sildenafil, some of which may be faster acting or even more efficacious. Down the road efficacious topical agents may also be developed. At some point, gene therapy will be made available and offer longer-term reversal of erectile dysfunction. The medical therapies will begin to move away from temporarily remedying erectile dysfunction to definitively curing the disorder. These prodigious research efforts are an outgrowth of the steady progress made in understanding the pathophysiology of erectile function.

Regarding the psychological aspects of erectile function, new theories are under investigation. For example, Bancroft and Janssen (1997) posit a dual-control system of sexual response predicated on central excitatory and inhibitory mechanisms. If confirmed, their findings may guide future psychological treatments.

While all of these ideas are exciting, clinicians must keep their eyes firmly on the mark—to remind themselves that although erectile function can be reduced to the molecular level, it remains an expression of the man's sexuality, and that it transpires in an interpersonal field where two people are exchanging love, passion, and intimacy with one another.

References

Aizenberg D, Zemishlany Z, Dorfman-Etrog P, et al: Sexual dysfunction in male schizophrenic patients. J Clin Psychiatry 56:137–141, 1995

Althof SE: Psychogenic impotence: treatment of men and couples, in Principles and Practice of Sex Therapy: Update for the 1990s. Edited by Leiblum SR, Rosen RC. New York, Guilford, 1989, pp 237–268

Althof S, Seftel AD: The evaluation and management of erectile dysfunction. Psychiatr Clin North Am 18:171–192, 1995

Althof SE, Turner LA: Self injection therapy and external vacuum devices in the treatment of erectile dysfunction, in Erectile Disorders: Assessment and Treatment. Edited by Rosen RC, Leiblum SR. New York, Guilford, 1992, pp 283–312

Althof SE, Turner LA, Levine SB, et al: Why do so many people drop out from auto-injection therapy for impotence? J Sex Marital Ther 15:121–129, 1989

Althof SE, Turner LA, Levine SB, et al: Long term use of intracavernous therapy in the treatment of erectile dysfunction. J Sex Marital Ther 17:101–112, 1991

American Psychiatric Association: Diagnostic and Statistical Manual of Mental Disorders, 4th Edition. Washington, DC, American Psychiatric Association, 1994

Annon JS: The Behavioral Treatment of Sexual Problems. Honolulu, HI, Kapiolani Health Services, 1974

Azadzoi K, Saenz de Tejada I, Goldstein I, et al: Characterization of rabbit corpus cavernosum in vitro. Surg Forum 39:640–641, 1988

Azadzoi KM, Kim N, Brown ML, et al: Endothelium-derived nitric oxide and cyclooxygenase products modulate corpus cavernosum smooth muscle tone. J Urol 147:220–222, 1992

Bancroft J, Jannsen E: The Kinsey Institute Model: some preliminary results. Paper presented at 23rd annual conference of the International Academy of Sex Research, Baton Rouge, LA, July 1997

Bodner DR, Lindan R, Leffler E, et al: The application of intracavernous injection of vasoactive medications for erection in men with spinal cord injury. J Urol 138:310–311, 1987

Brown SL, Hass CA, Koehler M, et al: Hepatotoxicity related to intracavernous pharmacotherapy with papaverine. Urology 52:844–847, 1998

Burnett AL, Lowenstein CJ, Bredt DS, et al: Nitric oxide: a physiologic mediator of penile erection. Science 257:401–403, 1992

Burnett AL, Nelson RJ, Calvin DC, et al: Nitric oxide dependent penile erection in mice lacking neuronal oxide synthase. Mol Med 2:288–296, 1996

Bush PA, Gonzalez NE, Ignarro LJ: Biosynthesis of nitric oxide and citrulline from L-arginine by constitutive nitric oxide synthase present in rabbit corpus cavernosum. Biochemical and Biophysical Research Communications 186:308–314, 1992

Christ G, Brink PR, Melman A, et al: The role of gap junctions and ion channels in the modulation of electrical and chemical signals in human corpus cavernosum smooth muscle. International Journal of Impotence Research 5:77–96, 1993

Christ G, Rehman J, Day N, et al: Intracorporal injection of hSlo cDNA in rats produces physiologically relevant alternations in penile function. Am J Physiol 275:600–608, 1998

Cooper A: Preliminary experience with a vacuum tumescence device (VCD) as a treatment for impotence. J Psychosom Res 31:413–418, 1987

DeAmicus L, Goldberg DC, LoPiccolo J, et al: Clinical follow-up of couples treated for sexual dysfunction. Arch Sex Behav 14:467–489, 1985

De Broe ME, De Backer WA: Pathophysiology of hemodialysis-associated hypoxemia. Adv Nephrol 18:297–300, 1989

Diedrichs W, Kaula N, Lue T, et al: The effect of subatmospheric pressure on the simian penis. J Urol 142:1087–1089, 1989

Eckardt KU, Kurtz A: The biological role, site and regulation of erythropoietin production. Adv Nephrol 21:203, 1989

Feldman HA, Goldstein I, Hatzichristou DG, et al: Impotence and its medical and psychosocial correlates: results of the Massachusetts Male Aging Study. J Urol 151:54–61, 1994

Garban H, Marquez D, Magee T, et al: Cloning of rat and human inducible penile nitric oxide synthase: application for gene therapy of erectile dysfunction. Biol Reprod 56:954–963, 1997

Goldstein I, Lue TF, Padma-Nathan H, et al: Oral sildenafil in the treatment of erectile dysfunction: Sildenafil Study Group. N Engl J Med 338:1397–1404, 1998

Gondre M, Christ GJ: Endothelin-1-induced alterations in phenylephrine-induced contractile responses are largely additive in physiologically diverse rabbit vasculature. J Pharmacol Exp Ther 286:635–642, 1998

Haas CA, Seftel AD, Razmjouei K, et al: Erectile dysfunction in aging: upregulation of endothelial nitric oxide synthase. Urology 51:516–522, 1998

Hawton K, Catalan J: Prognostic factors in sex therapy. Behav Res Ther 24:377–385, 1986

Hawton K, Catalan J, Faff J: Sex therapy for erectile dysfunction: characteristics of couples, treatment outcome, and prognostic factors. Arch Sex Behav 21:161–175, 1992

Heiman JR, LoPiccolo J: Clinical outcome of sex therapy. Arch Gen Psychiatry 40:443–449, 1983

Hricik DE, Schulak JA, Sell DR, et al: Effects of kidney-pancreas transplantation on plasma pentosidine. Kidney Int 43:398–403, 1993

Kifor I, Williams GH, Vickers MA, et al: Tissue angiotensin II as a modulator of erectile function; I: angiotensin peptide content, secretion and effects in the corpus cavernosum. J Urol 157:1920–1925, 1997

Kilmann PR, Milan RJ, Boland JP, et al: Group treatment of secondary erectile dysfunction. J Sex Marital Ther 13:168–182, 1987

Kim N, Azadzoi KM, Goldstein I, et al: A nitric oxide-like factor mediates nonadrenergic noncholinergic neurogenic relaxation of penile corpus cavernosum smooth muscle. J Clin Invest 88:112–118, 1991

Kim N, Vardi Y, Padma-Nathan H, et al: Oxygen tension regulates the nitric oxide pathway: physiological role in penile erection. J Clin Invest 91:437–442, 1993

Koreman S, Viosca S, Kaiser F, et al: Use of a vacuum tumescence device in the management of impotence. J Am Geriatr Soc 38:217–220, 1990

Krane RJ, Goldstein I, Saenz de Tejada I: Impotence. N Engl J Med 321:1648–1659, 1989

Levine S: Clinical Life: A Clinician's Guide. New York, Plenum, 1992

Levine S, Althof S: The pathogenesis of psychogenic erectile dysfunction. Journal of Sex Education and Therapy 17:251–266, 1991

Levine S, Althof SE, Turner LA, et al: Side effects of self-administration of intracavernous papaverine and phentolamine for the treatment of impotence. J Urol 141:54–57, 1989

Lewis R: Presented to the 8th World Congress on Impotence. Amsterdam, August 1998

Linet OI, Ogrinc FG: Efficacy and safety of intracavernosal alprostadil in men with erectile dysfunction: The Alprostadil Study Group. N Engl J Med 334:873–877, 1996

LoPiccolo J: Postmodern sex therapy for erectile failure, in Erectile Disorders: Assessment and Treatment. Edited by Rosen RC, Leiblum SR. New York, Guilford, 1992, pp 171–197

Lue TF, Tanagho EA: Physiology of erection and pharmacological management of impotence. J Urol 137:829–836, 1987

Masters WM, Johnson V: Human Sexual Inadequacy. Boston, MA, Little, Brown, 1970

Mohr DC, Beutler LE: Erectile dysfunction: a review of diagnostic and treatment procedures. Clin Psychol Rev 10:123–150, 1990

Monnier VM, Kohn RR, Cerami A: Accelerated age related browning of human collagen in diabetes mellitus. Proc Natl Acad Sci U S A 81:583–587, 1984

Mulcahy J: Overview of penile implants, in Diagnosis and Management of Male Sexual Dysfunction. Edited by Mulcahy J. New York, Igaku-Shoin, 1997, pp 218–230

Nadig P: Six years experience with the vacuum tumescence device. International Journal of Impotence Research 1:55–58, 1989

Nadig P, Ware J, Blumoff R: Noninvasive device to produce and maintain an erection-like state. Urology 27:126–131, 1986

National Institutes of Health: Consensus Development Conference Statement on Impotence. Bethesda, MD, National Institutes of Health, 1992

Nehra A, Goldstein I, Pabby A, et al: Mechanisms of venous leakage: a prospective clinicopathological correlation of corporeal function and structure. J Urol 156:1320–1329, 1996

Nonnast-Daniel B, Creutzig A, Kuhn K, et al: Effect of treatment with recombinant human erythropoietin on peripheral hemodynamics and oxygenation. Contrib Nephrol 66:185–194, 1988

Padma-Nathan H, Hellstrom W, Kaiser F, et al: Treatment of men with erectile dysfunction with transurethral alprostadil. N Engl J Med 336:1–7, 1997

Peroutka SJ: Endothelin receptors, in Handbook of Receptors and Channels: G-protein–coupled receptors. Edited by Peroutka SJ. Boca Raton, FL, CRC Press, 1994, pp 125–128

Rajfer J, Aronson WJ, Bush PA, et al: Nitric oxide as a mediator of relaxation of the corpus cavernosum in response to nonadrenergic, noncholinergic neurotransmission. N Engl J Med 326:90–94, 1992

Reynolds B: Psychological treatment of erectile dysfunction in men without partners: outcome results and a new direction. J Sex Marital Ther 2:136–145, 1991

Rosen RC, Leiblum SR: Erectile disorders: an overview of historical trends and clinical perspectives, in Erectile Disorders: Assessment and Treatment. Edited by Rosen RC, Leiblum SR. New York, Guilford, 1992, pp 3–26

Rosen RC, Leiblum SR, Spector IP: Psychologically based treatment for male erectile disorder: a cognitive interpersonal model. J Sex Marital Ther 20:67–85, 1994

Rosen R, Goldstein I, Heiman J, et al: A Process of Care Model: Evaluation and Treatment of Erectile Dysfunction. Piscataway, NJ, Robert Wood Johnson Foundation, 1998

Saenz de Tejada I, Blanco R, Goldstein I, et al: Cholinergic neurotransmission in human corpus cavernosum: responses of isolated tissue. Am J Physiol 254:459–467, 1988

Saenz de Tejada I, Kim N, Lagan I, et al: Regulation of adrenergic activity in penile corpus cavernosum. J Urol 142:1117–1121, 1989

Schnarf D: Constructing the Sexual Crucible. New York, WW Norton, 1990

Seftel AD: Molecular Urology 3:103–107, 1999

Seftel AD, Viola KA, Kasner SE, et al: Nitric oxide relaxes rabbit corpus cavernosum smooth muscle via a potassium-conductive pathway. Biochemical and Biophysiological Research 219:382–387, 1996

Seftel AD, Vaziri ND, Ni Z, et al: Advanced glycation end products in human penis: elevation in diabetic tissue, site of deposition and possible effects through iNOS or eNOS. Urology 50:1016–1026, 1997

Segraves RT: Antidepressant induced sexual dysfunction. J Clin Psychiatry 43:48–54, 1998

Sell DR, Monnier VM: Isolation, purification and partial characterization of novel fluorophores from aging human insoluble collagen rich tissue. Connect Tissue Res 19:77–92, 1989

Sidi A, Cameron JS, Dykstra DD, et al: Vasoactive intracavernous pharmacotherapy for the treatment of erectile impotence in men with spinal cord injury. J Urol 138:539–542, 1987

Sidi A, Pratap R, Chen K: Patient acceptance of and satisfaction with vasoactive intracavernous pharmacotherapy for impotence. J Urol 140:293–294, 1988

Simonsen U, Prieto D, Delgado JA, et al: Nitric oxide is involved in the inhibitory neurotransmission and endothelium-dependent relaxations of human small penile arteries. Clin Sci 92:269–275, 1997

Simonson MS, Kester M, Baldi E, et al: Endothelins: renal and cardiovascular actions. Adv Nephrol 21:177–194, 1992

Tiefer L, Melman A: Comprehensive evaluation of erectile dysfunction and medical treatments, in Principles and Practice of Sex Therapy: Update for the 1990s. Edited by Leiblum SR, Rosen RC. New York, Guilford, 1989, pp 207–236

Turner LA, Althof SE, Levine SB, et al: Self-injection of papaverine and phentolamine in the treatment of psychogenic impotence. J Sex Marital Ther 15:163–176, 1989

Turner LA, Althof SE, Levine SB, et al: Treating erectile dysfunction with external vacuum device: impact upon sexual psychological and marital functioning. J Urol 144:79–82, 1990

Turner LA, Althof SE, Levine SB, et al: Long term use of vacuum pump devices in the treatment of erectile dysfunction. J Sex Marital Ther 17:81–93, 1991

Vardi Y, Saenz de Tejada I: Functional and radiologic evidence of vascular communication between the spongiosal and cavernosal compartments of the penis. Urology 49:749–752, 1997

Virag R, Shourky K, Fluoresco J, et al: Intracavernous self injection of vasoactive drugs in the treatment of impotence: 8 year experience with 615 cases. J Urol 145:287–292, 1991

Williams G, Abbou C, Amar E, et al: Efficacy and safety of transurethral alprostadil therapy in men with erectile dysfunction. Br J Urol 81:889–894, 1998

Witherington R: Vacuum tumescence device for management of erectile impotence. J Urol 141:320–322, 1989

Zentgraf M, Ludwig G, Ziegler M: How safe is the treatment of impotence with intracavernous autoinjection? Eur Urol 16:165–171, 1989

Zilbergeld B: The New Male Sexuality. New York, Bantam, 1992

Chapter 4

Fatherhood as a Transformation of the Self: Steps Toward a New Psychology of Men

William S. Pollack, Ph.D.

> *If I am not for myself, who will be for me?*
> *And if I am for myself alone, then what am I?*
> *If not now, then when?*
>
> Hillel

Centuries ago the Jewish sage Hillel's existential plea for a balance between an investment in the self and a connection with or a commitment to others—a balance between the sense of an "I" and a "We"—foreshadowed our modern day, gender-based struggles concerning autonomy, affiliation, and intimacy. Although many men, like their women counterparts, have come to intellectually accept the necessity for a type of emotional interdependence in life, the deepest personal meanings of their dependent needs are often experienced as a frightening anathema to men. The poet John Donne advised in the 17th century, "No man is an island, entire of itself; every man is a piece of a continent, a part of the main. . . . Any man's death diminishes me, because I am involved in mankind. . . . Therefore never send to know for whom the bell tolls; it tolls for thee."

Yet most modern men continue to function emotionally much more akin to Robert Frost's neighbor in the poem *Mending Wall*, who felt that "good fences make good neighbors." Men are often found walling themselves off from their own feeling states, fending off sadness, depression, and empathic intimate relationships in ways that cause their significant others to feel a great deal of pain and consternation and, I would argue, in ways that often tend to hurt and confuse the men themselves.

Traversing the path that leads to parenthood is, for many men, an arduous journey. Becoming and being a father presents men with a challenge much akin to the duality represented by the Chinese ideograph for change: CRISIS/OPPORTUNITY. The crisis is found in the "unfinished business" and long-buried unconscious struggles from childhood that threaten to become dramatically unearthed; and the opportunity is found in life's greatest second chance—to father in a new way that both transforms our selves and leaves a legacy of paternal nurturance for the next generation.

Fatherhood, then, may function as a transformation of the male-engendered self. In turn, our acknowledgement of men's significant role in parenting must prod us to transform our own psychoanalytically informed developmental psychology as it concerns boys' normative growth and men's emotional health. Although we have always taken for granted in psychoanalysis that we know what men want, recent developments in the study of women's lives and the type of data presented today about fathering force us to rethink this "male question." I hope it will also propel us toward the first steps in a new psychoanalytic psychology of men.

Almost 20 years ago, Michael Lamb (then a pioneer researcher on the impact of fathers on their children's lives), decried the academic wasteland in which men's contributions to family life had gone unheralded and unstudied. In 1975 he called fathers "the forgotten contributors to child development" (Lamb 1975). It was many more years before we came to realize how the experience of becoming a father was a forgotten contribution to men's development. Perhaps that was because our developmental models focused so narrowly on early childhood and were so woefully inadequate when it came to late adolescence and adulthood. I believe it was also because we had so championed the ideal of autonomy and separation, especially in "normal" men's development, that we neglected to understand the significance of affiliative attachments in male psychological health. As a result, we overlooked the powerfully transforming role of becoming a father. Indeed, the shock of how men's nurturant urge—often suppressed in boyhood and adult socialization tasks—can be stimulated by becoming a father is one of the most joyous discoveries surrounding men's experience of paternity (Greenberg and Morris 1974).

For example, Jerry, a man whose progress to fatherhood we observed in the Boston University Pregnancy and Parenthood Project,[1] expressed, in a poignant and articulate response to our interview, this joyous shock and the subsequent psychological changes wrought by becoming a father:

> It has been a lot of fun to watch her grow, but at the same time it is a lot of responsibility. . . . I just had never been around babies, and I didn't know. I just didn't have any idea of what being a father was all about. . . . And I am really attached. I find myself thinking about her at work, rushing to the day-care center to pick her up, just because every day she learns something new, and you just want to see it and kind of share it with her.
>
> My personality has changed a lot. I take things a little slower. I think about her more. I guess when you decide to have a baby, you don't think about those things. You don't think your life is really going to change. All of a sudden, you've got to be somebody's father! It is different, but it's fun.

John, another man struggling with his new fathering role, made manifest the ambivalence inherent in taking on such a nurturant responsibility versus one's own self (sometimes called narcissistic) needs:

> Well, it's difficult for me to live with anyone. . . . I could spend a great deal of my time alone. Without having a wife . . . without

---

[1] The Boston University Pregnancy and Parenthood Project was a longitudinal study under the direction of Francis K. Grossman. The work on father autonomy and affiliation was done by William Pollack in collaboration with Dr. Grossman and his colleagues Dr. Ellen Golding and Nikki Fedele (Pollack 1982, 1983; Grossman et al. 1987; Grossman et al. 1980; Pollack and Grossman 1985).

having children. But, at the same time, all those things are very important to me. . . . If I could be 100% selfish and just have my wife when I wanted her and just have my kids when I wanted to—that would suit me. But I can see that marriage wouldn't last. So it becomes a . . . balancing act, a constant balancing act. Between her needs, my needs, and the child's needs.

Rethinking Development: Men and Women

Research has begun to show that a man's need to cling to independence at the cost of intimacy seems driven by emotional imperatives that begin in boyhood. As feminist scholars (e.g., Chodorow, Gilligan, Miller) have pointed out, girls and boys develop quite differently. Girls are generally encouraged to maintain their closeness to their mother, whereas boys are usually pushed to make a more clear-cut separation. Received psychoanalytic wisdom has held that boys are expected to "disidentify" (Greenson 1968) from their mothers. That is, they are expected to become intrapsychically separate in order to become appropriately identified as masculine.

Early Development

Chodorow (1978, 1989) asserted that because women are still largely responsible for caregiving in the early years of a child's life, the consequent issues of gender identity formation differ in critical ways for boys and girls. For girls, identity formation will occur through the integration of, or identification with, an ongoing relational attachment to the mother. For boys to define themselves as masculine, they must be different. There must be a more clear-cut separation from the mother, both intrapsychically and interpersonally. Maintenance of this sense of separateness and difference may require a defensive hardening of the self and ego boundaries of little boys and, later, of adult men—on both conscious and unconscious levels.

According to Chodorow, this process has a socially constructed basis and may change as childrearing patterns shift. Until that occurs, differential developmental processes of nurturance will generally propel men and women in different directions. If one accepts Chodorow's argument, one must basically agree with her that "because women mother, the sense of maleness in men differs from the sense of femaleness in women" and masculinity (or maleness) becomes more conflictual, and more problematic, than femaleness:

> Underlying, or built into, core male gender identity is an early, non-verbal, unconscious and almost *somatic sense of primary oneness with the mother, an underlying sense of femaleness that continually, usually unnoticeably but sometimes consistently challenges and undermines the sense of maleness.* Thus, because of the primary oneness and identification with his mother, a primary femaleness, a boy's and man's core gender identity . . . is an issue. (Chodorow 1989, p. 109, emphasis added)

What becomes clear, from this perspective, is that little boys and grown men are unconsciously needing to fend off an earlier sense of oneness with their mother—which tends to threaten their gender identity and independent sense of self. Girls "grow up with a sense of continuity and similarity to their mother, a relational connection to the world," whereas boys do not have this opportunity. Because of both the historical childrearing practices that create the significance of the mother and the consequent "absence of concrete, real, available male figures of identification and love who are [equally] salient" for the boy, "learning what it is to be masculine comes to mean learning to be *not* womanly." As a result, separateness becomes more salient for boys than for girls. Boys and, later, men tend to eschew feminine identifications and experiences such as dependency, strong feelings, and relational bonding.

Beyond Freud—Beneath the Oedipus Complex

Although Freud and his early followers linked core sexual and gender identity to the crucible of the Oedipus complex and its resolution, it has become clear that core gender identity issues (i.e., the sense of masculinity) emerge much earlier than this in a child's psychic development. Deep in the adult man's psyche lies the formative experience of a little boy, struggling to maintain a sense of a masculine self, vis-a-vis his attachment to his mother. He is also struggling with the very real loss of an earlier affiliative oneness, which can never be regained—within this model—without a threat to masculine identity.

Although Chodorow's discussion of gender identity development is insightful, it does not adequately capture what this experience of development must feel like for a little boy. The emphasis remains on the bond between mothers and daughters. Nowhere do we get a sense of the loss associated with the boy's definition of his own identity and core gender self: an experiential process that requires separation from the most cherished, admired, and loved object in his life—at what would be an inappropriate time from the point of view of girls' development. Equally significant, this broken maternal connection or "disidentification" (Greenson 1968) occurs within a social context of childrearing in which 1) girl siblings are allowed to remain connected and 2) the father often remains absent or emotionally unavailable to his young son, as an alternate nurturing figure for the "lost" mother.

A Normative (Gender-Linked) Developmental Trauma

Chodorow (1978, p. 166) suggests that the intrapsychic developmental events so significant to the young boy may be played out reciprocally and interpersonally between mother and son: "though children of both sexes are originally part of her self, a mother *unconsciously* and often *consciously* experiences her son as more of an 'other' than her daughter. Reciprocally, a son's male core gender identity develops away from his mother." This is more than just a subtle emotional shift. It is akin to a behavioral push:

> Mothers tend to experience their daughters as more like, and continuous with themselves. . . . By contrast, mothers experience their sons as a male *opposite*. Boys are more likely to have been *pushed out of the pre-oedipal relationship* and to have had to curtail

their primary love and sense of empathic tie with their mother. A boy has been engaged *and been required to engage* in a more emphatic individuation and a more defensive firming of experienced ego boundaries. (Chodorow 1978, p. 166, emphasis added)

As a consequence of this behavioral "push," males may be more vulnerable than females to traumatic and premature separations—disruptions that may later be experienced by the child as a loss or abandonment.

I have argued (Pollack 1992) that we may be seeing a developmental basis for a gender-specific vulnerability to traumatic abrogation of the early holding environment, an impingement in boys' development—a normative life-cycle loss—which may, later in life, leave many adult men at risk for fears of intimate connection. This traumatic experience of abandonment occurs so early in life that the shameful memory of the loss would likely be repressed deeply.

Not only do boys have a more problematic course toward identity, but they also have a continuing need to defend against urges toward affiliation and intimacy, because of the repressed trauma of shameful and premature separation. This is a loss that ensued with their mothers and that was often unassuaged as a result of their father's inability to assume an alternative nurturant role. Having experienced both a sense of hurt in the real connection to their mothers (as a result of her societally constructed role to make gender differentiation clear) and the subsequent loss of finding no equally salient alternative in their fathers, many boys and, later, men are left at risk for empathic disruptions in their affiliative connections.

Later relationships may revive the deeply repressed yearnings toward the early mother. The result may be the creation of transitional or self-object relationships with mother substitutes that are meant to both repair and assuage the unspeakable hurt of premature, traumatic separation and to deny simultaneously the loss of the relational bond. In their unconscious yearning for closeness, men may seek out women who meet their needs—only to deny them any mutually empathic response, in order to protect themselves from the fears or dangers of reexperiencing the repressed pain, sadness, or depression that affiliation now conjures. Such men maintain that they are self-sufficient, while they are in the midst of an interdependent connection itself. This paradox, combined with women's reasonable expectation that the significance of their relational capacities be recognized, may lead to much of the misunderstanding seen in the traditional, intimate relationships that men and women form. It also accounts for much of the pain experienced by men and women, as they attempt to listen to and interpret one another's "voices" (Gilligan 1979, 1982). Elsewhere I have argued that this paradox may account for the preponderance of males with the diagnosis of narcissistic personality disorder and for the requirement, in the treatment of this disorder, of what Modell calls the symbolic actualization of the holding environment or what Kohut defines as the stabilizing self-object transference.

The Balancing Act: The "I" and the "We"

Although much of the revisionist critique of developmental theory has continued to focus on the different pathways for men and women along the axes of independent identity—aloneness (i.e., autonomy) versus connectedness (i.e., affiliation), bifurcated along gender lines (Chodorow 1978, 1989; Gilligan 1979, 1982), there is reason to suspect that a balance (within each gender) between the capacity for I-ness and We-ness (following George Klein's concepts) is a better predictor of mental health and of the capacity to sustain intimate relationships (Klein 1976; Pollack 1982, 1990, in press). The findings of the Boston University Parenthood and Pregnancy Project (BUPP) provide empirical support for a model of healthy emotional development for adult men that requires a gender-specific balance between the capacities for autonomy and affiliation, between separateness and relatedness—that is, between I-ness and We-ness.

The BUPP was a longitudinal developmental study of 90 couples first seen while the women were pregnant with the indexed children. Women were interviewed alone close to the beginning of their pregnancy (half of the women were pregnant with a first child) and with their husbands later in the gestational period.

Each family (i.e., mother, father, and indexed child) was studied at the child's birth and when the child was 1, 2, and 5 years of age. Data were collected during home visits and using naturalistic and structured observations, semistructured interviews, paper-and-pencil scales, and child assessments. Researchers used standardized clinical ratings derived from interaction observations, videotaped and audiotaped segments of play, and interviews in conducting complex time-linked statistical analyses. (Details of the larger study may be found in Fedele et al. 1988, Grossman et al. 1980, and Pollack and Grossman 1985.) Among the issues explored were the transition from nonparent to parent, the marital couple's needs and satisfaction, the men's and women's changing sense of self, the children's affective and cognitive functioning and development, the quality of parenting, and general family adaptation (Fedele et al. 1988; Grossman et al. 1987; Grossman 1987, 1988; Pollack and Grossman 1985; see also Pollack, in press).

Among the strongest findings from the BUPP was that parents' autonomy and affiliation scores (more specifically, the achievement of a healthy balance between autonomous functioning and affiliative relatedness) were predictive of marital satisfaction, "good-enough" fathering (discussed in detail later in this chapter), parenting capacity, the children's positive mood, and family adaptation (Grossman et al. 1987, 1988; Pollack 1982, 1983, 1989; Pollack and Grossman 1985). These findings are in contrast to traditional views of autonomy as an alternative to, or as the opposite of, affiliation and relatedness (Erikson 1963). The perspective offered here is one of a dialectic (Grossman et al. 1988; Pollack 1990): autonomy is related to but not defined solely by participation in separate activities, and affiliation is not just a matter of engaging in relationships. Gerald Stechler and Samuel Kaplan (1980), two child psychoanalysts who built on Klein's work, defined the beginning sense of self in children and its later integrated form in adults as a combination of two apparently disparate aspects that must be integrated into one identity. They conceptualized two poles within one cohesive self: the first is experienced as an autonomous center of activity, and the second is experienced as part of a transcendent unit. They called the autonomous pole the "I" component and the more affiliative pole the "We" component. I agree with Stechler and Kaplan that the self can be experienced as separate and simultaneously as part of an entity greater than itself. In our research, when we talk about autonomy we are referring to the sense of the "I" within the self, and when we talk about affiliation we are referring to the sense of the "We" embedded within an independent self (Grossman et al. 1988; Pollack 1982).

Although the autonomy-affiliation balance was important for both women and men, men's definition of what was affiliative and what was autonomous differed radically from women's. Any attempt to measure these two concepts required awareness of these basic differences. For example, the men in the study would often show a strong proclivity to be close to their children but would express this by attention, physical play, or teaching. Women appeared to be more comfortable in holding and hugging their children. We felt that both types of interaction indicated affiliative capacities, which the children's responsiveness corroborated (Pollack and Grossman 1985).

Given the unique nature of men's affiliative interactions, we needed to develop gender-specific scales to measure these constructs. Not merely an artifact of one empirical study, this finding has been replicated by other prominent research groups studying empathy (Hoffman 1977; Lennon and Eisenberg 1987), substantiating the gender-specific nature of such concepts as self-sufficiency, warmth, empathy, relatedness, and so on (Pollack 1982, 1983). Rather than creating a rigid gender-linked dichotomy between capacities for self-sufficiency (I-ness) and relatedness (We-ness) (i.e., the independent man versus the interdependent woman), the empirical data suggest a basis for recasting these functions along the lines of a balance. The data also indicate that at times there may be a "his" relatedness and a "hers" relatedness, and a "hers" autonomy and a "his" autonomy. Men's mental health and psychological well-being, then, are not reflected solely in achieving autonomy but rather are a balance between relatedness and independence. Fatherhood both upsets that balance and offers opportunities for its realignment.

Fatherhood: A Second Chance

In reviewing our research from the BUPP, we found several major trends in healthy couples' negotiations about parenting. For example, in a traditional family structure (in which women take on the primary role of child care), men shy away from competing with this role of primacy with the children. I am not talking here about a dysfunctional setting in which women feel stuck with their children and men are off doing something else. Rather these couples decided on such an emotional division of labor for their mutual benefit and needs. When something goes wrong in this setup (e.g., the mother becomes ill or incapacitated), the father is more than ready to step in, give support, and take on an alternative nurturant function. We described this balance as one of *complementarity*. Perhaps such complementarities need to be renegotiated at times, and the possibilities of excluding the man from emotional connection, or abandoning the woman to too much, need to be addressed. Such an arrangement can continue to allow the father a significant role in parenting—meaningful for child and mother—even though it may not always be the leading role.

Sometimes unconscious expectations based on deeply ingrained gender roles may impede fathers from taking up their new task of parenting. The mother could become an inadvertent gatekeeper, keeping her newborn baby from her husband. This happens in usually subtle ways. For example, the mother might hand the baby to the father at an inopportune moment and then say, "Oh, dear, don't hold her like that," or "That isn't the way to change a diaper." Often the father, who already felt inadequate, would unconsciously collude by hastily giving the baby to his wife and then backing off. With men and women increasingly invading each other's traditional turf, it is understandable that women may feel inclined to maintain some control over the household, especially over parenting.

On the father's side, we noticed a parallel unconscious process, which I've called nest-feathering, occurring around the time of the child's birth and continuing into the child's first year. The new father often felt that the best way to provide for his wife and child was to work assiduously in order to gain greater income or career status—to "feather the nest," in which the young fledgling and his or her caring mother were placed. What most distressed the women in the study was the emotional absence of their husbands while they were pregnant. Much like the O'Henry story "The Gift of the Magi," the husband was sacrificing for the wife, and the wife for the husband, in ways that were terribly out of sync.

Our advice to these new fathers was that they spend some of their time supporting their wife and newborn by being physically and emotionally present. We suggested to their wives that they try to help their husbands learn how to take care of the newborn. We believe that men need to accept that their wives can mentor them in some nurturing skills. At the same time, they also need their wives to recognize that "male" ways of parenting can be a valuable complement to mothering.

We also found an important result concerning the effect of the quality of the father's time on their interaction with the children. All parenting research has shown that many fathers spend an extremely small period of their day with their children, even if they are "highly" involved (Grossman et al. 1988). Our findings showed that the quantity and quality of the time need not be the same. In other words, fathers in our study who were highly involved with their work and were satisfied with that work (i.e., spending a fair amount of time at it) could not spend equal amounts of time with their children. However, the quality of the time that these "job-satisfied fathers" spent with their children directly and positively affected their children's mental health. A word of caution must be stated here: I am not saying that fathers can abandon their families and the quality of connection will be the same. Rather, in the families that we studied, work-invested fathers who care about their children and spend significant time with them—albeit not the same amount of time as the mothers do—can still have an important effect on the emotional well-being of their children—because of the quality of the interaction. Fathers, even those who are actively at work, do count and do make a big difference. Even if men are not the primary caregivers, they may have an important effect on the mental health of their families and children and, by extension, on themselves. Often this represents a second chance for a reparative relationship and, via this repair, for an enhanced sense of intimacy for themselves, their mates, and their families.

A trend was noted in the interviews of men who were found to be healthy supporters of both autonomy and affiliation in their children. These men stated that they were invested in learning how to parent correctly and learned to do so not only from their own memories of parental nurturance but also from the direct observation of their wives. These men often considered their wives as parenting experts and observed their wives so that they could learn to be good parents themselves. We understood this trend to be a form of identification for the men. This process offers another chance for repair, especially in the couples' situation. For men, being able to value the tasks that women do traditionally, particularly in mothering and child care—and to identify with these nurturing roles—helps to undo at the deepest unconscious layers the fear and dread that many men feel about being dependent on a woman (Pollack, in press). Perhaps it begins to undo the psychic damage wrought by a forced *disidentification* from early maternal love objects.

Good-Enough Fathering: Fathering as a Developmental Phase

Fathering is one of men's greatest opportunities for personal transformation (Betcher and Pollack 1993). The psychoanalyst Theresa Benedek (1959, 1975) created the term *fatherliness*, by which she meant an instinctually rooted trait that is characterized by empathic responsiveness to one's children. She believed fatherliness originated in the man's earliest psychic memory traces of mother and father. Although Benedek's work was groundbreaking, I prefer the term *good-enough fathering*, adapted from a term that Winnicott (1974) used for mothers (Diamond 1992; Pollack and Grossman 1985). This term encompasses the biological capacities of fatherhood and the more far-reaching, overarching social and intrapsychic constructions of fatherliness that Benedek described. It also addresses the father's capacity to be both progenitor and protector, not only distantly as a food gatherer, hunter, and warrior, but also proximally as nurturant caregiver, within a monogamous family system.

For two reasons, I wish to extend good-enough fathering beyond the close-touch world of caring for one's own children. First, a father who cares only for his own child but cares little about other children in the world cannot possibly inculcate the kind of reparative experience in his family and in himself that was lost for many men in premature separation from a loving connection. This capacity must go beyond selfishness, beyond a narrowly defined family loyalty. Second, there are many men who for one reason or another will never have the opportunity to experience being a father to their own children. Yet there is no reason that this capacity for good-enough fathering cannot emerge within them and be expressed by them. I am referring to a concept that is closest to Erikson's sense of *generativity*: a caring supportive mentoring type of role to younger "others," which the nurturant older man experiences as a type of good-enough parenting.

Becoming a man should not entail a single rigid pathway but rather a multitude of possible journeys toward fulfillment. Men and women become trapped when the personality characteristics necessary for mature involvement in our complex industrialized world become divided along gender lines. It is no more useful for men to be protectors and providers without the capacity for deep empathic feeling or for sharing sadness with their mates, than it is for women to be nurturing caregivers to children but be denied the capacity for achievement at work.

Fathering is a powerful emotional role for men. Although research has tended to focus on the absence or loss of the father, the presence of the father and the normative experience of fathering lie at the deepest emotional roots of men's psychosocial being. The BUPP findings have been corroborated by a number of other innovative interventions (Barnett et al. 1992; Levant 1990) and indicate that good-enough fathering is not only a salient factor in the healthy development of young boys and girls but is an important curative or transforming factor in the mental health of adult men.

Contrary to past and popular belief, fatherhood is as signifi-

cant to many men as is career achievement. It appears to have a re-
verberating impact on their emotional capacities for balance,
mental health, and physical well-being. Barnett et al. (1992) found
that the quality of men's "parental role" was a significant factor in
their psychological distress or health and concluded, "The
widely held belief that men's psychological health is primarily
determined by their work role is . . . deficient; the quality of
men's family roles contributes strongly to their mental health"
(p. 366). Barnett and Marshall (1991) found that for married fathers the only factor significantly correlated with their physical
health was the quality of their relationships with their children.
There was no correlation between the health of these men and
their work or marital role. Robert Bly poetically sums up this
transformational matrix:

> . . . and slowly the kind man comes closer, loses his rage,
>   sits down at table.
> So I am proud only of those days that pass in undivided
>   tenderness,
> when you sit drawing, or making books, stapled, with
>   messages to the world,
> of coloring a man with fire coming out of his hair.
> Or we sit at a table, with small tea carefully poured.
> So we pass our time together, calm and delighted.

> (Bly 1986; "For My Son Noah, Ten Years Old")

Based on the results of the BUPP study, I have suggested that,
for two reasons, men's capacity to achieve a gender-sensitive empathic form of fathering provides the opportunity for a transformation of men's self-structure. First, men can recognize the
positive effect of their emotional commitment on the well-being
of their children—both girls and boys. Men are now able to give to
their children something that often they did not receive from their
own fathers (Pollack, in press). This altruistic transformation
broadens men's ego ideal and, therefore, enhances their capacity
for self-esteem. In addition, it often requires identifying with and
internalizing their wives' caregiving capacities, at times learning
how to nurture from their female partners. In so doing, men are

acknowledging the meaningfulness of women's relational skills and are reinternalizing this positive sense of maternal caregiving in a manner that can dramatically repair the earlier renunciation and splitting off of all aspects of the self deemed feminine and maternal.

Personal Transformations

The men in the BUPP study were by and large not very positive about the role model that their own fathers had provided for them as parents. Primarily they had aspirations to be better fathers to their own children than their fathers had been to them. They felt that their own mothers had been good parents, and they used that maternal nurturant experience and their identification with their wives' caregiving skills to make up for whatever gaps they felt existed in their own paternal self-image.

Most of the men in the BUPP study responded in the negative to questions about whether they thought they were the same kind of father to their children that their own father had been to them and about whether they felt more like their own father now (i.e., since becoming a father). "Definitely *not*," exclaimed one man. "No. I feel *less* like him, more conscious of the threat of being like him," answered another father who had felt quite hurt by his own father's parenting. "I don't know if my father was that great a father. I'd like to be a better father," he added (Grossman et al. 1980).

When we asked John, a man who we followed up throughout the transition to parenthood, whether he felt more like his father since becoming one, his answer reflected the active psychological process of achieving a balance between accepting a legacy from the past and creating a new experience in the present:

> Well, in respect to being a father, I am not the same kind of father. But being a father, yes I feel more like him now than I ever did before. . . . [I]t is different, it's sort of a mystical thing that I can't explain that . . . well . . . but it creates a sort of bond between my father and myself when I see my children growing up. Because for the first time I'm getting a feeling for what he must have felt while I was growing up.

By the end of his child's first year, John was saying that he enjoyed "helping with the diapering" and being an active co-parent with his wife. When asked whether there were differences between what a father and mother could do with an infant, he replied:

I don't mind getting involved with taking care of him in general. But the relationship is obviously not the same. He sees his mother, you know, and until yesterday she was breast-feeding him for a whole year, so there's another attraction between the two of them. I couldn't have, I wish I could, but couldn't have that type of relationship with him. When he looks at me, he smiles, but it is not the same sort of smile he flashes to his mother.

Indeed, John was able to admit that he was jealous of this special relationship but that it was just something he had to accept. He was equally aware of how becoming a father had started to have profound effects on his own personality:

Well, I have to face up to the fact that I'm going to be 35 years old and have to start acting like that, because to a certain extent, inside, I still feel like I'm 10 years old, and I want to go out and play baseball or do things like that . . . I think that it has added a lot of responsibility, much of which I have accepted begrudgingly. But sometimes I feel like getting in my car and driving away and, you know, doing anything that a single person would do . . .

By the time of his baby's second birthday, John was aware of a significant shift in his personality structure:

I think I've become a little more responsible and—obviously—I spend more time thinking of my family than I do about myself. I would say when I was first married I spent a great deal of time thinking about myself and then probably about my wife . . . and now I think my priorities—well it's my family instead of myself. I still treat myself pretty well, but my priorities have changed.

Part of these changes in sense of self reverberate with an enhancement of self-esteem that accrues when a man spends time at home and dedicates himself to his child:

> I think I'm pleased with myself that I have lived up to the responsibility of being, in my opinion, a good parent. I didn't know that about myself (before), and I definitely had questions about whether or not I would handle it.

When asked whether he would think of himself as a member of his family first or as an individual first, he replied quite quickly: "Definitely I would say a member of my family first."

When John's child was 5 years old, John reflected on the fact that slowly but surely he had become "more generally concerned with my family and the quality of the home life as opposed to how well I'm going to do in my profession." He thought this was a painful choice—at times "very upsetting"—but felt on the whole "more satisfied than if I had done it the other way and spent the time trying to achieve some success outside of the house." His acceptance of this "daddy track" was a quiet one; he still felt that when he needed to deny a client's request for time, he had to make up an excuse that was along the lines of a doctor's or dentist's appointment rather than letting the client know that he really wanted to go to his son's little league game.

John had gone from being "100% selfish" through a "balancing act" to having his role as a father become the most important thing in his life. Having achieved a personal transformation, he felt now that he was part of a larger community or life cycle beyond himself. In tackling our questions about the ways that having a child reminded him of his own childhood, John waxed eloquent about his personal experience of how the child is father to the man and the man is father to the child of the next generation:

> Probably the most vivid [experience] in my mind was last week. I happen to love the beach. I can remember [vividly], probably from the time I was 3 years old, the feeling of sitting on the warm sand, feeling the warm sun and breeze, and playing in the sand . . . , as if it happened 15 minutes ago. And last year I had John, Jr., on the beach, and he was sitting at the same spot, roughly, that we sat on 30 years ago.
> Yes, the same street, the same beach, and I was looking at him, typical little Greek-looking kid with dark curly hair and a fat

stomach, which is what I probably looked like, and I got shocked, scared out of my wits. Because, I was . . . sitting here, Jesus Christ, 30 years ago, and I was sitting there . . . watching myself, and that was a really scary afternoon. I mean it was nice, but it was pretty unsettling. Realizing that I was pretty near halfway.

Halfway through the life cycle, he meant, but fully transformed through the experience of fathering. But what happens when men are less able to allow themselves the experience of becoming a father?

Inhibitions and Interruptions in the Transition to Fatherhood

The following vignette illustrates some of the inhibitions or psychological interruptions that may make it difficult or impossible for certain men to experience becoming a father. The vignette illustrates the possibility of achieving the psychological growth necessary to embrace fatherhood at any point in the life cycle (even several years after the child's birth) and, as such, illustrates the distinction between merely being a father and developing what Benedek (1959, 1975) called fatherliness.

Today it is not atypical for modern men with career aspirations to delay fathering until later in life, and the term "late" father is usually reserved for men who have a child later in the life cycle. Here I use the term to note a more striking shift: the capacity to take on true fathering responsibilities later in the life of one's child.

A "Late" Father

Arnie was a successful business executive in his mid-50s when he first sought psychological consultation. His stated reason for seeking treatment was the apparent impending dissolution of his 20-year marriage to his childhood sweetheart. Arnie reported all of the pain that had developed in the last 3 years of the marriage, including a growing emotional isolation from his wife and an inability to share his feelings with her. Arnie had had a series of extramarital affairs, in order to deal with what he called a sense of boredom or deadness in the marriage. During the last affair, his wife confronted him and he admitted everything—including his growing despair that the marriage was leading nowhere and that he might need to leave. Arnie's wife was distraught by the possibility that he was being unfaithful to her and by the reality that he might seek a divorce. She sought psychotherapeutic advice and suggested that he do the same.

Arnie was not reluctant to enter therapy, but he questioned whether it could "really do me any good." He felt that his problems "went way back" and that his style of behavior, including the use of extramarital affairs, was something he had "just gotten used to." The early treatment sessions consisted of history taking and focused on the "here and now" explosions that took place in the marriage and continually threatened to lead to premature resolution, prior to deeper therapeutic comprehension.

The therapist was getting only a shadowy sense of Arnie's own relationship with his father and, in turn, of Arnie's relationship with his now 10-year-old daughter, Rachel, so he inquired first about the father-daughter pair. Arnie quickly responded that he had never talked about Rachel in therapy because he didn't think it had "anything to do with why I was here." On further elaboration, it became clear that he was quite alienated from his daughter and felt that she was "my wife's child." Because of some perinatal difficulty, Rachel had required around-the-clock interventions as a young infant, which were administered mostly by Arnie's wife—as he was often at work 60–70 hours per week. From then on, Arnie explained, "I felt like I lost the opportunity to really be Rachel's father," as his wife became an active, autonomous, and primary parent. "I didn't really know what to say to her," Arnie explained. As a result, he often withdrew, leaving Rachel and her mother to "do their own thing."

As he spoke more about his estrangement from his daughter, Arnie appeared sad, and the therapist pointed out this affective shift. Arnie agreed that perhaps for a long time he had hidden from himself how much he missed this father-daughter relationship. The therapist then asked whether something was being repeated here that Arnie had experienced as a child with his own father.

The floodgates opened. Arnie remembered how abandoned he had felt as a younger child and again as an adolescent when he had sought his father's support. Because of a series of business setbacks, and the abrupt onset of a psychiatric illness, his father was totally unavailable to him in anything but a cold, cognitive manner. Arnie remembered how much he kept trying to "please him" but to no avail. Arnie's father died when Arnie was in his early 20s, and he remembered feeling only "relieved that I didn't have to try to get his love anymore."

Arnie, who had already begun a trial separation from his wife before starting treatment, arranged for visitation periods with his daughter. He realized that even though his contact with his wife would be minimal during this trial period, he wanted to maximize his connection with Rachel. He set up periods during the week and over the weekend in which they would do things by themselves. Sometimes they would get together as a family.

Returning to therapy several weeks later, Arnie was beaming with pride. He explained, "I think I'm spending more time with Rachel and more quality time than when I lived at home." Indeed, this did not seem like denial or distortion but rather a true expression of the shift in the parenting relationship. Arnie asked, "I don't have to be like my own father, do I?" Without waiting for the therapist to answer, Arnie replied for himself, "No! I don't." He added, "Maybe I'm fooling myself, but I think, divorce or not, I'm creating a much closer relationship with Rachel, and I don't feel that will be lost."

Although the marital difficulties continued, Arnie felt that he had worked through a very important piece of his personal experience, concerning the earlier pain and disappointment with his own father. He felt that only now, just before his daughter's 10th birthday, had he, for the first time, become a father to his daughter. Just as Mahler has commented on the "psychological birth of the infant," there is an equally important point in time that we might call the "psychological birth of the father." Although optimally it will occur while awaiting the birth of the child, there is no reason why a capacity for fatherliness cannot be generated, with psychotherapeutic intervention, at any point in the parent-child life cycle. Such intervention may address inhibition resulting from unconscious conflicts or deficits in the father's own experience of parenting as a child.

What Do Men (and Boys) Really Need?

Fathering, then, forces us to reformulate the question "What do males want?" as "What do boys and men really need?" I am suggesting that our psychoanalytic (and, by extension, psycho-dynamic) conceptual models of gender development have done boys and girls and men and women a disservice: by hopelessly confusing the binary bedrock of *core gender identity* (i.e., being male or female) with the more elastic diversity of *gender role alternatives.* Although core gender identity happens very early and offers few choices, gender role identity, or identification, is a much more complex concept or process—representing the internalization of unconscious psychic schemas of what "being a man" or "being a woman" means to a particular individual, mediated by the context of the individual's own society, culture, or family. As I have argued in my book on the present crisis in boys' development (Pollack 1998), we must free males from gender straitjackets. Then we would expect to see the widest range of healthy alternatives or engendered identities (including so-called heterosexual and homosexual object choices), unless a culturally rigid set of standards attempts to channel such normal diversity into a limited set of societally acceptable norms. If the latter happens, we are likely to experience—as we have unfortunately seen during the past century—the utilization of psychoanalysis (a creative theory of unconscious dynamics and human development) as the handmaiden for reductionistic, essentialist views of masculinity and femininity. This leads to the muddling of social constructs with biological givens and the use of the heuristic findings of a developmentally based science as a repressive social tool for conformity.

Feminist critics such as Chodorow (1978, 1989) and Miller (1976) have rightfully taken to task our phallocentric models of identity (read: men = healthy; women = dependent/sick). The replacements offered, while appropriately elevating women's bonded or relational selves to a high level of significance, continue to support unwittingly a gender-bifurcated and essentialist model of nurturant girls versus unempathic boys, self-in-relation women versus self-sufficient men. Such a model redresses the imbalance of the power dialectic but maintains a traditional set of gender distinctions.

I suggest that we must go beyond this point to lay the foundations of a new psychoanalytic theory of gender development and identity. We must create a paradigm that integrates the best elements of psychoanalytic models of unconscious internalization (an empathic developmental psychology) with state-of-the-art knowledge of biological processes and the necessary hermeneutic of an interpersonal and social construction of meaning.

Men are struggling to be decent and responsible. Men are struggling to exist in connection with women and with other men without fear. A new psychoanalytic psychology of men and boys—a reframing or transformation of masculinity—would recognize the heroic effort inherent in such a struggle.

We must replace the fanciful and grandiose notions of heroic fathers from afar with the painful realities and sweet successes of everyday paternal life. Barbara Ehrenreich, in writing a critique of the so-called "new man," states:

> So it is not enough, anymore, to ask that men become more like women; we should ask instead that they become more like what *both* men and women *might* be. My new man, if I could design one, would be capable of appreciation, sensitivity, intimacy—values that have been for too long, "feminine." But he would also be capable of commitment, to use that much-abused word, and I mean by that commitment not only to friends and family, but to a broad and generous vision of how we might all live together (1990, p. 137).

Conclusion

Why is it that we live in an age in which fathers' contributions to children's development are finally recognized, but the salient role of being and becoming a nurturant, caring father remains relatively unexamined in its centrality to men's own emotional health and development? The continued overemphasis by our society on the autonomous ("I") component of the psychological makeup of little boys and, later, adult men has not only taken its toll on intimate relationships (Pollack 1998), but it has too often kept men from achieving a true sense of emotional paternity—one that balances the autonomy of self with the affiliative capacity of connections.

True fathering is a balancing act: a balance between the urge to achieve independently and the equally pressing need to be connected to meaningful others, beyond one's self. It is a balance between men's often less-than-complete experience of nurturing caregiving from their own fathers and their opportunity for achieving a different model of fathering for the next generation and—through this struggle to change—achieving a personal, psychological transformation for themselves. The journey to fatherhood is often a challenging one, at times fraught with impediments; however, these impediments can be overcome as men become more in touch with the inner world of feelings and with the shadowy, unconscious repository of our childhood world of play and pain. The ultimate balance that fathering may offer men is one between the day-to-day exigencies of adult life and the wellspring of inner life that paternal nurturance must—by its very existence—tap into. A poem by the psychoanalyst Donald Winnicott is a fitting evocation of the inner balance that fathering can bring to men, when men can safely and positively come to fathering:

> Let down your tap root
> To the center of your soul
> Suck up the sap
> from the infinite source
> of your unconscious
> And
> Be evergreen

Men can be aided in this process by a new gender-aware psychoanalytic psychology and by clinicians' enhanced empathic understanding that men's defenses often reflect a traumatic dilemma requiring an affective bridge to greater connection (Pollack and Levant 1998). Then men may leave their walled-off islands of defensive self-sufficiency and slowly and carefully build bridges of intimacy to the mainland. If so, we may see not only more empathically balanced, stable, engendered selves but also the creation of a more flexible set of internalized self and object relations—balanced between the "I" (autonomy) and the

"We" (affiliation)—a set of repaired fathering connections, benefiting men and all those who love them. In the opening words of the sage Hillel, "If not now, then when?"

References

Barnett RC, Marshall NL:Physical symptoms and the interplay of work and family roles. Health Psychology 10:94–101, 1991

Barnett RC, Marshall NL, Plick JH: Men's multiple roles and their relationships to men's psychosocial distress. Journal of Marriage and the Family 54:358–367, 1992

Benedek T: Parenthood as a developmental phase: its contribution to the libido theory. J Am Psychoanal Assoc, 1959, pp 389–417

Benedek T: Discussion of "Parenthood as a Developmental Phase." J Am Psychoanal Assoc, 1975, pp 154–165

Betcher W, Pollack WS: In a Time of Fallen Heroes: The Re-creation of Masculinity. New York, Atheneum, 1993

Chodorow N: The Reproduction of Mothering. Berkeley, CA, University of California Press, 1978

Chodorow N: Feminism and Psychoanalytic Theory. New Haven, CT, Yale University Press, 1989

Diamond MJ: Creativity in becoming a father. Journal of Men's Studies 1:41–45, 1992

Ehrenreich B: The Worst Years of Our Life. New York, Harper, 1990

Erikson EH: Childhood and Society. New York, WW Norton, 1963

Fedele NM, Golding ER, Grossman FK, et al: The adult-to-parent transition: psychological issues in adjustment to first parenthood, in Current Theory and Research on the Transition to Parenthood. Edited by Michaels GY, Goldberg WA. Cambridge, England, Cambridge University Press, 1988

Gilligan C: Woman's place in men's life cycle. Harvard Educational Review 49:365–378, 1979

Gilligan C: In a Different Voice. Cambridge, MA, Harvard University Press, 1982

Greenberg M, Morris N: Engrossment: the newborn's impact upon the father. Am J Orthopsychiatry 44:520–531, 1974

Greenson RR: Dis-identifying from mother: its special importance for the boy. Int J Psychoanal 49:370–374, 1968

Grossman FK: Separate and together: men's autonomy and affiliation in the transition to parenthood, in Father's Transition to Parenthood. Edited by Berman P, Pedersen FA. Hillsdale, NJ, Erlbaum Associates, 1987, pp 24–39

Grossman FK, Eichler LS, Winickoff SA, et al: Pregnancy, Birth and Parenthood. San Francisco, CA, Jossey-Bass, 1980

Grossman FK, Pollack WS, Golding ER, et al: Autonomy and affiliation in the transition to parenthood. Family Relations 36:263–269, 1987

Grossman FK, Pollack WS, Golding E: Fathers and children: predicting the quality and quantity of fathering. Dev Psychol 24:82–91, 1988

Hoffman ML: Empathy, Its Development and Prosocial Implications. Nebraska Symposium on Motivation. Lincoln, University of Nebraska Press, 1977

Klein G: Psychoanalytic Theory. New York, International Universities, 1976

Lamb ME: Fathers: forgotten contributors to child development. Hum Dev 18:245–266, 1975

Lennon R, Eisenberg N: Gender and age differences in empathy and sympathy, in Empathy and Its Development. Edited by Eisenberg N, Strayer J. Cambridge, England, Cambridge University Press, 1987, pp 195–217

Miller JB: Toward a New Psychology of Woman. Boston, Beacon Press, 1976

Pollack WS: "I"ness and "We"ness: parallel lines of development. Unpublished doctoral dissertation, Boston University, 1982

Pollack WS: Object-relations and self psychology: researching children and their family systems. The Psychologist-Psychoanalyst 4:14, 1983

Pollack WS: Boys and men: developmental ramifications of autonomy and affiliation. Paper presented at the midwinter meeting of the American Psychological Association Division of Psychotherapy, Orlando, FL, February 1989

Pollack WS: Men's development and psychotherapy: a psychoanalytic perspective. Psychotherapy 27:316–321, 1990

Pollack WS: Should men treat women? dilemmas for the male psychotherapist: psychoanalytic and developmental perspectives. Ethics and Behavior 2:39–49, 1992

Pollack WS: Real Boys: Rescuing Our Sons From the Myths of Boyhood. New York, Random House, 1998

Pollack WS, Grossman FK: Parent-child interaction, in The Handbook of Family Psychology and Therapy. Edited by L'Abate L. Homewood, IL, Dorsey, 1985, pp 586–622

Pollack WS, Levant RF: New Psychotherapy for Men. New York, Wiley, 1998

Stechler G, Kaplan S: The development of the self: a psychoanalytic perspective. Psychoanalytic Study of the Child 35:85–106, 1980

Winnicott DW: The Maturational Processes and the Facilitating Environment. New York, International Universities Press, 1974

Chapter 5

Casualties of Recovered Memory Therapy: The Impact of False Allegations of Incest on Accused Fathers

Harold I. Lief, M.D., and Janet M. Fetkewicz, M.A.

A false accusation of childhood sexual abuse may become such a defining feature of a man's life that it remains salient, even after death, as in the case of Chicago's Cardinal Bernardin. In 1993 the Cardinal was accused of sexual abuse by Peter Cook, a former seminarian, who reportedly recalled the abuse under hypnosis. Eventually Cook retracted his accusations, realizing that his memories of sexual abuse at the hands of the Cardinal were false. Cardinal Bernardin died in 1996. Reports of his death and stories about his life as a religious leader were numerous, and many mentioned the public accusations of sexual abuse (Steinfels 1996; Woodward and McCormick 1996).

False accusations of childhood sexual abuse levied against fathers based on the recovery of memories during therapy have been a topic of growing interest, as attested by the increasing number of professional publications, the vast amount of media attention, and the steadily mounting number of lawsuits, even criminal charges, against therapists, including psychiatrists (*United States of America v. Peterson et al.*). The impact of false accusations on the family and the pain and anguish created have been reported (de Rivera 1994; Goldstein and Farmer 1992; Pendergrast 1996), but scarce attention has been paid to the psychology of the fathers accused. In this chapter, we explore the effect of false allegations of incest on men who are accused. We focus on accusations by adults based on newly "recovered" repressed memories of childhood sexual abuse.

There is a clear distinction between victims of sexual abuse with continuous memories and adults who recover new memories of childhood sexual abuse. We should not confuse these two groups of individuals. Much of the emotionalism and the politicization of the recovered memory debate is a result of the blurring of these lines. The blurring of the two groups is not restricted to the popular press. It also occurs in the professional literature. An example of this confusion is found in the research of Herman and Schatzow (1987), who reported that in a group of 53 incest survivors, 74% (39 of 53) were able to locate corroborating evidence of their memories. This study is often used to demonstrate the validity of newly recovered memories of incest in adult survivors. But as Brenneis (1997) points out, the bulk of verification presumably came from 39 women who had never forgotten the incestuous experiences. Fourteen women were apparently fully amnesic, but it is impossible to tell how many of those women were able to corroborate their memories with external evidence. As Brenneis notes, "In addition, the members of the fully amnesic subgroup are depicted as obsessed with doubts about the reality of their suspected early incestuous experience" (p. 58).

There is no debate about the real problem of sexual abuse, which can have a severe psychological impact on survivors. Most survivors carry around the memories of their traumatic experiences. These individuals should receive the best care that the therapeutic community has to offer. Those who recover new memories of sexual abuse should also receive the best care. It is our hope that the professional community can discuss and refine standards for assessment and treatment of both groups, recognizing both the damage caused by genuine sexual abuse and the damage of false accusations.

Lief summarizes this notion: "While our awareness of childhood sexual abuse has increased enormously in the last decade and the horrors of its consequences should never be minimized, there is another side to this situation, namely that of the consequences of false allegations where whole families are split apart and terrible pain inflicted on everyone concerned. This side of the story needs to be told, for a therapist may, with the best intentions in the world, contribute to enormous family suffering" (Sifford 1991, p. F1).

False allegations of sexual abuse have implications not only for the accused parent (usually the father) but also for the spouse, other children, and extended family. Family relationships are reconfigured, and the accusation becomes a defining feature of those relationships. A family's struggle occurs within the broader context of the debate about false memories and false accusations of childhood sexual abuse. We will discuss this phenomenon from a social, historical, and psychological perspective and pay special attention to the psychology of the fathers accused. Toward this end, we conducted a series of interviews with fathers whose accusing daughters had recognized their recovered memories of sexual abuse as false and retracted their accusations.

Overview

The debate over the accuracy of newly recovered memories of childhood sexual abuse continues to rage. This discussion rests on central questions surrounding memory mechanisms and recovered memories of sexual abuse: 1) Can memories of chronic childhood sexual abuse be repressed completely? 2) If so, can those memories be recovered? 3) Are there special clinical techniques that are effective tools in recovering repressed memories? 4) Once memories are recovered, how is their accuracy determined? Differences in beliefs and practices among mental health professionals will determine their responses to these questions.

Repression

During the 20th century, the concept of repression seems to have been taken for granted by the majority of psychiatrists. Is it a workable hypothesis that is more helpful than hurtful? If it is an invalid hypothesis, should it not be abandoned? Is reliance upon repression as an organizing concept of therapy questionable at best?

Holmes (1990) reviewed the research on repression and was unable to find any study that supported the validity of the theory of repression. More recently, Pope et al. (1998) reviewed prospective studies of documented survivors of trauma and their memories of the traumatic experiences. They found no evidence that subjects developed dissociative amnesia for, or repressed, traumatic events. Although recent reports have purported to demonstrate the documented existence of amnesia for childhood sexual abuse (e.g., Scheflin and Brown 1996), careful examination of the data reveals substantive methodological weaknesses that yield questionable conclusions (Piper 1996).

In response to the controversy over scientific evidence for repression, the *Diagnostic and Statistical Manual of Mental Disorders,* Fourth Edition, in its discussion of dissociative identity disorder and other dissociative disorders, shifted from the term "repression" to "dissociative amnesia." The theory is that trauma, especially childhood trauma, creates a brain process leading to a dissociative episode, in which explicit memories of the trauma are lost. Although the name of the mechanism has changed, the approach to the buried memories remains the same. According to theorists and clinicians, the original memories can be retrieved through the use of recovered memory therapy (RMT), especially if the clinician pays attention to the emerging implicit memories—which take the form of bodily sensations (often called "body memories"), repetitive behaviors, flashbacks, and so on.

Recovery of Memories

If memories of childhood sexual abuse can be repressed, can they be recovered? A positive response to this question relies on several related assumptions:

1. That memories of childhood sexual abuse are somehow "special," that is, they *can* be recovered accurately and are not subject to the vagaries of normal memory (i.e., change, decay, confabulation)
2. That the "carriers" of these repressed memories can somehow be identified, that is, certain symptoms, behaviors, or

psychopathology identify a survivor of sexual abuse before he or she has access to the repressed memories of the abuse
3. That some technique, or collection of techniques, is an effective tool in the recovery of accurate memories

These assumptions have been discussed elsewhere (Lindsay and Read 1994; Loftus 1993; Pope and Hudson 1995). The consensus is 1) that there is no evidence for special features of memories of incest, 2) that mechanisms proposed to explain the absence of abuse memories such as repression and dissociation are vague and have a wide range of definitions, 3) that symptom profiles have been so diffuse and contradictory that they are unreliable as identifiers of victims of sexual abuse, and 4) that many of the techniques thought to be effective tools to unearth repressed memories can also result in false impressions with heightened confidence in them on the part of the patient (Garry et al. 1996; Perry 1995).

Professional organizations have issued statements cautioning their members about some of the beliefs and techniques associated with RMT (American Medical Association 1994; American Psychiatric Association 1993; American Psychological Association 1995; Australian Psychological Society Limited 1994; Brandon et al. 1997; Canadian Psychiatric Association 1996). For example, the American Psychiatric Association (1993) states, "[C]are must be taken to avoid prejudging the cause of the patient's difficulties, or the veracity of the patient's reports. A strong prior belief by the psychiatrist that sexual abuse, or other factors, are or are not the cause of the patient's problems is likely to interfere with appropriate assessment and treatment." A stronger statement has been issued by the Royal College of Psychiatrists in its consensus recommendations for practice: "Psychiatrists are advised to avoid engaging in any 'memory recovery techniques' which are based upon the expectation of past sexual abuse of which the patient has no memory" (Brandon et al. 1997).

Although it is unlikely that the debate will end any time soon, there seems to be agreement that false accusations of sexual abuse can and do occur (although there is argument over the prevalence). Some researchers and clinicians (e.g., Karlin and Orne

1996; Lindsay and Read 1995; Yapko 1994) maintain that false diagnosis of a history of sexual abuse (and therefore false accusations of abuse) is more prevalent than currently assumed.

False Memory Syndrome

The cases that we discuss in this chapter involved a reported false accusation and subsequent recantation of sexual abuse. Most documented cases follow a similar pattern: an individual enters psychotherapy; he or she has no reported history of childhood sexual trauma; and over time, and often through the use of suggestive techniques by the therapist, the individual comes to believe that he or she was sexually abused in childhood and, further, that the abuse was an etiologic factor in his or her current symptomatology. This belief often has a dramatic impact on the patient's view of himself or herself, on the accused, and on other family members.

A definition of false memory syndrome has been offered by Kihlstrom (1998, p. 16):

> A condition in which a person's identity and interpersonal relationships are centered around a memory of a traumatic experience which is objectively false but in which the person strongly believes. Note that the syndrome is not characterized by false memories as such. We all have memories that are inaccurate. Rather, the syndrome may be diagnosed when the memory is so deeply ingrained that it orients the individual's entire personality and lifestyle, in turn disrupting all sorts of other adaptive behavior.

The processes and implications of the development of pseudo-memories have been examined by a number of authors (de Rivera 1997; Lief and Fetkewicz 1995; McElroy and Keck 1995; Nelson and Simpson 1994). These authors have examined those elements from the perspective of individuals who "recovered" false memories and later relinquished their memories as inaccurate. These individuals are often referred to as *retractors,* or recanters. Some retractors have published first-person accounts of their experiences with false memories (Gavigan 1992;

Goldstein and Farmer 1993; Pasley 1994). There is a newsletter written by retractors and a Web site on the Internet.

Studies and anecdotal reports of the experience of individuals who recovered pseudo-memories have been consistent in their explication of this experience. Most of the subjects of these reports are women who entered therapy with a variety of presenting problems such as depression, relational difficulties, anxiety, or life stressors (e.g., birth, death, divorce). Retractors report that current factors, perhaps reflected in their presenting problems, were not a focus of treatment; rather, treatment became a search for a causal relationship between the presenting problem and re-pressed childhood sexual abuse (Loftus and Ketchum 1994; Ofshe and Watters 1994; see also Lindsay and Read 1994; Pendergrast 1996). For example, in a survey of 40 retractors, Lief and Fetkewicz (1995) found that over 82% of these subjects re-ported a direct suggestion by their therapist that childhood incest was the cause for their current distress, when no such experience had been reported to the therapist.

Retractors report that the search for memories became the cor-nerstone of therapy while the therapist played an increasingly dominant role in the life of the patient. One subject conveyed this urgency and the deepening dependent transference that fueled it: "I was concerned that I had no memories yet, so I pressured my-self to start remembering. I had a feeling that my therapist would scold me or be disappointed in me if I didn't remember some-thing. I was scared not to remember . . . " (Lief and Fetkewicz 1995, p. 423). Some authors have compared this type of therapeu-tic relationship to cult-like behavior, in which devotion to and de-pendency on the therapist are the emotional hallmarks (Goldberg 1997).

The therapy described by retractors often included the use of techniques to exhume or, as one writer referred to it, "liposuc-tion" (DuChateau 1998) buried memories of sexual abuse. These techniques include hypnosis, guided imagery, age regression, Amytal interviews, group therapy, and self-help literature. When memories did surface, they most often involved sexual abuse by a father. Half of the cases in one survey included accusations of a dramatic nature (e.g., involving satanic ritual abuse) (Lief and

Fetkewicz 1995). In at least one popularly prescribed reading for many retractors, a psychologist writes that indicators of an emerging memory may include "anxiety, inexplicable depression, nightmares . . . an increase in self-abusive behavior" (Frederickson 1992, p. 184). After memories emerge, she cautions, "full-blown delayed post-traumatic stress disorder appears. . . . Depression either sets in or worsens . . . you feel hopeless" (Frederickson 1992, p. 216). Our own research confirms that most patients become worse as a consequence of this form of therapy (Fetkewicz et al., in press; Lief and Fetkewicz 1995).

Theoretical Issues

It is important to recognize how much RMT has in common with the theoretical underpinnings of psychoanalysis. RMT is based on the theory that patients' presenting problems (e.g., depression, marriage problems, eating disorders) can be explained by the fact that they have repressed memories of traumatic sexual abuse. The belief that psychological trauma leads to a walling off from consciousness of memories and the emotions accompanying the trauma—which, in turn, accounts for psychic or bodily symptoms and maladaptive behavior patterns—is not a new idea, peculiar to RMT. This, precisely, was the theory propounded by Freud, strongly influenced by his observations of Charcot, in his early studies of hysteria. This schema is still a cornerstone of psychoanalytic theory, albeit modified by more sophisticated theories about self psychology and debates about the nature—indeed, the very existence—of repression or its most recent relation, dissociative amnesia. Controversial in 1898, and yet again in 1998, is the nature of trauma. At first Freud believed, allegedly based on the words of his patients, that actual sexual abuse had taken place in childhood. When he gradually realized that these were not historically accurate memories but were false, or pseudo-memories as we would call them today, he set forth the notion that the "trauma" was the patients' unconscious sexual fantasies that had arisen in childhood, directed toward a parent.

Freud abandoned his original ideas about historically accurate memories of childhood sexual abuse, not because "of the fear of criticism," as Masson (1984) has charged, but because he gradually recognized that he was influencing patients' recollections. Later, he seems to have "forgotten" the role of his own influence on the productions of his patients and denied that suggestion takes place in psychoanalysis (Freud 1938/1964).

Role of Suggestion

Despite Freud's denials, his method was one in which he would suggest an idea (an "interpretation") to his patient and then, under the influence of this suggestion, retrieve more and more associations substantiating his hypothesis. The correctness of the analyst's construction of the puzzle (as in a jigsaw puzzle) relies on the elicitation of additional associations that "fit" in completing the puzzle and on whether the patient accepts the truth of the construction. Although Freud believed that he had abandoned direct suggestion when he abandoned hypnosis, it is clear that suggestion, both direct and indirect, was and remains a key element in psychoanalysis. In addition to direct suggestion, there are extraordinary influences based on the expectations of the therapist. These expectations provide indirect or implicit suggestions. Freud apparently believed that this did not take place, saying that free association guaranteed to a great extent that nothing would be introduced into psychoanalysis by the expectations of the analyst (Freud 1946). In this connection, Marmor (1970) writes "clinical experience has demonstrated that this simply is not so and the free associations of the patient are strongly influenced by the values and expectations of the therapist" (p. 161). In addition to the kind of questions asked in face-to-face transactions, the expression on the therapist's face, a questioning glance, a lift of the eyebrows, and a barely perceptible shake of the head or shrug of the shoulder all act as significant cues to the patient. "But even *behind* the couch our 'uh-huhs' as well as our silences, the interest or the disinterest reflected in our tone of voice or our shifting posture all act like subtle radio signals influencing the patient's responses, reinforcing some responses and discouraging others. That this influence actually occurs has been confirmed experimentally by numerous observers" (p. 161). Marmor continues, "As a result, depending on the point of view of the psychoanalyst, patients of every psychoanalytic school tend, *under free association,* to bring up precisely the kind of phenomenological data which confirm the theories and interpretations of their analysts! Thus, each theory tends to be self validating" (p. 161).

Mutually Reinforcing Beliefs

In the transaction between the therapist and the patient, agreement by the patient is taken as proof of the correctness of the interpretation or the construction. Paradoxically, if the patient disagrees, it is also taken as proof that the construction is correct. The disagreement is proof of the power of the walled-off impulse, fantasy, or memory, and it is called *resistance.* There is no sure way to differentiate between resistance and genuine disagreement. In RMT, disagreement is termed *denial;* in satanic ritual abuse cases it is often attributed to the work of a satanic cult, an external agency, causing the patient to clam up.

In RMT, the evolution of pseudo-memories also depends on suggestion, both explicit and implicit. Many of the retractors we studied reported that the therapist made a direct suggestion, such as "Your stories and symptoms fit the idea that sexual abuse is likely, or very likely to have occurred to you in your childhood" (Lief and Fetkewicz 1995). The therapist may make a somewhat less direct suggestion by implying that some trauma occurred in childhood, and because sexual abuse is in the popular press, films, and television, the patient is primed to wonder if the trauma was sexual abuse. The therapist may believe that he or she is neutral yet reinforces the idea in the nonverbal ways described by Marmor (1970). Constructions by the patient are often accepted as factual memories. Brenneis (1997) states, "A powerful mutually reinforcing loop, based more on process than substance, may be created" (p. 46).

Once the idea either is implanted or develops spontaneously in the patient and is reinforced by the therapist, circularity becomes a central feature of the therapist-patient relationship. As the patient brings in more and more material, it seemingly documents the correctness of the idea. The therapist is increasingly convinced of the accuracy of the original proposition and presents his or her reinforced views to the patient, who provides still more material for substantiation, and so on. Like all positive feedback systems that operate without brakes, it tends to spin out of control. Often, in RMT, more perpetrators are named, more incidents are remembered, more alters come to the surface, and more horrors are added (in satanic ritual abuse cases) until the entire drama becomes so unreal, or the patient becomes so sick, that better reality testing finally becomes the brake that halts the system. Reality testing often takes place only when excessive amounts of prescribed psychoactive medications are decreased or there is a complete separation from the therapist.

In the therapeutic relationships discussed by retractors, reinforcement of suggestion often occurs when the therapist offers rewards for bringing up additional associations (Lief and Fetkewicz 1995). For example, if the therapist is pleased by the new material, he or she may give the patient privileges for being a good patient. Similarly, the therapist may use threats (e.g., of being sent to a locked hospital unit) in response to the failure to recover new memories. Reinforcement of suggestion also occurs through reading material that the therapist may suggest (e.g., *The Courage to Heal* [Bass and Davis 1988]) and through the films shown in some dissociative disorder units in mental hospitals (e.g., *Sybil, Rosemary's Baby*). Groups play a large role in this reinforcement and the atmosphere of contagion (reminiscent of Charcot's patient groups), as there is a sense of celebration as new "memories" are reported to the group.

In a study of nonclinical subjects, Mazzoni et al. (Mazzoni GAL, Lombardo P, Malvagia S, Loftus EF: "Dream Interpretation and False Beliefs," unpublished manuscript, 1997) demonstrated the power of dream interpretation as a clinical intervention. In simulated therapy sessions, subjects were given a suggestion that their dreams indicated an event in their past (having been lost before the age of 3 years). Even though these same subjects had reported no such remembrance from their past, they adopted the false belief suggested by the therapist's interpretation of their dream. The authors ask the question: "Are therapists aware of the power they have?" If Mazzoni et al. found that nonclinical subjects could be influenced to develop a false belief about their past, a vulnerable, distraught therapy patient who looks to the therapist as an authority on his or her problems may be even more suggestible.

Therapeutic Assumptions

Freud's "talking cure" was based on the theory that for the cure to take place, repressed material had to be made conscious. Although there is little evidence that these early patients were helped by abreaction or catharsis, therapy aimed at retrieving repressed memories persisted over the past century. During World War II, for example, psychiatrists used hypnosis and intravenous Pentothal or Amytal to recreate battle experiences, allowing patients to discharge accompanying emotions. Psychiatrists were never certain whether such experiences per se, or the contrast between them and the safe environment in which they were reenacted, were the helpful agents.

These theories about the cause and cure of psychopathology were still "in play" in 1980 when the RMT movement began to accelerate. The following social forces came together at about that time:

1. A growing awareness of the extent of child sexual abuse, which led to the development of child-protection organizations and institutions (many of which were governmental) and to the passing of laws in most states mandating that health professionals report suspected child abuse
2. A society that embraced the notion of victimization
3. The self-help or recovery movement—a consequence of the "culture of complaint" (Hughes 1993), representing an attempt to cope with the status of "victim" and characterized by group therapy for every conceivable distress from A to Z (i.e., from alcoholism to zoophobia)
4. Radical or "gender" feminism (Sommers 1994). (One would think that feminists would eschew the notion of inevitable

gender-related weakness, but the perceptual mindset of the powerful, often evil male was a more dominant influence.)

The conjunction of these social forces and the prevailing theories about the causes and cures of psychogenic mental illness created the RMT movement. Hundreds, probably thousands, of therapists seized upon it as the capstone of psychotherapy. Surveys of Ph.D. therapists indicate misinformation about the nature of memory, hypnosis, and trauma among respondents (Poole et al. 1995; Yapko 1994). For example, Yapko (1994) found that over half (54%) of the clinicians surveyed believed that hypnosis can be used to recover memories from as early as birth, almost half (43%) believed that scant memory of childhood is indicative of trauma, 41% believed that memories from the first year of life can be recovered, and one third (33%) endorsed the notion that the mind records events like a computer.

The belief that childhood sexual abuse was the root cause of so much adult misery had a number of obvious advantages:

1. It was a parsimonious explanation, a simplistic reduction of complex phenomena.
2. It could shift the blame from the patient to external causes.
3. It could use a simple formula for cure.
4. It could create a strong bond and almost impregnable therapeutic alliance between patient and therapist (i.e., "us against them").

These advantages became magnified if the patient were diagnosed with multiple personality disorder (now called dissociative identity disorder), which was frequently associated with satanic ritual abuse. The pace of this social and mental health development can be seen in the number of cases of multiple personality disorder. Shorter (1992) commented on the rise and fall in the prevalence of this disorder. For example, it was less commonly diagnosed in 1950 than in 1900, when it was a fashionable diagnosis. It reemerged in the 1980s, with thousands of cases subsequently diagnosed and numerous dissociative disorders units formed in mental hospitals. Now many of these units have been closed.

Impact of an Accusation

Paul Ingram, a religious family man and a sheriff in Olympia, Washington, was accused of horrific abuse by his daughters (Wright 1994). His disbelief of these accusations was overwhelming, and in fact, no abuse had occurred. He was shocked and incredulous that his daughters would accuse him falsely. After hours of interrogation, Ingram confessed to abusing his daughters, saying, "I really believe that the allegations did occur and that I did violate them and probably for a long period of time. I've repressed it. . . . They wouldn't lie about something like this" (Wright 1994, p. 8).

Of course, Ingram's reaction was atypical. Most fathers express complete incredulity at accusations of incest. The first response for many men is to question their own innocence and search their souls for any indication that this could have occurred, for example, by asking themselves, "How could my beloved child accuse me, if it's not true?" Sometimes fathers consider the possibility that, if they did not commit incest, they must have done something wrong and attempt to determine what that might be, with the hope that all will be explained and resolved.

Researchers have conducted several large surveys of families in which there was an accusation of sexual abuse by an adult child (M. Elson, unpublished manuscript, 1998; False Memory Syndrome Foundation 1997; Freyd et al. 1993; Goodyear-Smith et al. 1997; Gudjonsson 1997). These surveys obtained data in several broad areas, including demographics, information about family life, events surrounding the accusation, and information about the accuser. In general, families were similar across surveys in terms of age, ethnicity, socioeconomic status, and level of education. The families surveyed tended to identify themselves as predominantly Caucasian, middle class, and well educated. Accusers in all surveys are typically female, with above-average educational achievement. Accusers typically grew up with both parents, in intact families, and parents tended to remain married after the accusations. The events surrounding the accusations also indicated similar patterns. The memories on which the accusations were based were recovered in therapy; in most cases, the use of controversial techniques to recover memories (e.g., hypnosis, Amytal interviews) was reported; the alleged abuse was thought to have been chronic and often initiated in early childhood; and in 15%–20% of the cases, accusations included satanic ritual abuse. Only one survey (False Memory Syndrome Foundation 1997) included a subset of families in which there had been a retraction ($n = 144$ of a total $N = 2056$). Data were reported as comments from these families. For example, "After five years of hell, my daughter retracted," and "It's all like a bad dream now."

Although the impact of allegations of sexual abuse on the accused father was not the focus of these surveys, some of the surveys addressed related factors. For example, M. Elson (unpublished manuscript, 1998) questioned families about changes in mental, physical, and emotional health after the accusation. In this sample ($n = 83$), 96% of the respondents reported a deterioration in general health and psychological health. Complaints included depression, nightmares, suicidal ideation, severe stress reaction, impotence, and anger. Although a direct causal connection between the accusation and these complaints cannot be asserted, respondents felt strongly that the stress of the accusations and estrangement from their accusing daughters had an enormous impact on their well-being.

Accused fathers interviewed by Pendergrast (1996) discussed reactions of confusion, anger, bitterness, hurt, compassion, grief, and loss. Some fathers maintain that it is "best" to be accused of extreme abuse, such as satanic ritual abuse, because the outrageousness of the accusations makes them less believable by others. The worst, others claim, is to be accused by more than one child because the father cannot rely on assertions of his innocence by his other children.

De Rivera (1994) interviewed nine couples who faced an accusation of sexual abuse by an adult child. In eight of the nine cases, the accused was the husband—the father of the accuser. The interviews focused on factors of interest to us: the responses of the spouse of the accused and of the accused himself, the impact on the marriage, the family's "management" of the situation, the emotional support obtained by the accused, and the coping mechanisms used.

In de Rivera's sample, the most common emotional reactions of the accused parent included pain, anger, and "bouts of uncontrollable crying" (1994, p. 151). De Rivera points out that the management of anger is crucial and concludes that the feelings of rage expressed by these subjects, coupled with helplessness in the face of such an accusation, can result in depression. One possible coping style is "shutting down," that is, avoiding thinking about the accusation, but most of the interviewees tended to channel their anger into working toward resolution.

De Rivera found that the spouses' most typical reactions were shock and confusion: does a wife believe her child or trust in her husband? As one spouse reported, "I was frantic. It couldn't be true . . . but what if it were . . . ? He's not the type. . . . But my children don't lie" (de Rivera 1994, p. 150). The wives interviewed by de Rivera eventually came to believe their husbands. He maintains that four factors influenced this shift from questioning to believing:

1. The memories are "logically inconsistent" with factual information.
2. The primary reactions of the husband are emotional pain and consistent denial of the accusations.
3. The wife realizes that she could not have overlooked ongoing abuse and cannot reconcile her part in the accuser's narrative.
4. The possibility existed that the accuser was influenced in therapy, which seems a more logical explanation for the accusations.

Another source of information about the impact of false allegations on the accused is the growing number of legal cases in which retractors and parents are co-plaintiffs in lawsuits against therapists. For example, in three such legal cases that have been resolved—one by a jury verdict for the plaintiffs and the others by settlement—excerpts from parents' causes of action indicated a range of complaints including emotional distress, damage to family relationships, and damage to reputation:

- *Marietti et al. v. Kluft et al.:* As a result of the defendant's treatment, the parents alleged negligent infliction of emotional distress, intentional infliction of emotional distress, slander, and loss of consortium. The complaint states that the parents underwent great shock and mental anguish and experienced loss of affection and alienation in their family relations.
- *Althaus v. Cohen:* The parents in this case were criminally charged and suffered the obvious consequences of a criminal investigation. Causes of action against the therapist included negligence and invasion of privacy.
- *Fultz v. Carr and Walker:* In this case the parents were the in-laws of the retractor. They stated that, as a result of the defendant's negligence, they suffered mental anguish, damage to their reputations, and prolonged separation from their grandchildren.

Interviews With Accused Fathers

Method

The False Memory Syndrome Foundation[1] maintains a database of families who report a false accusation of sexual abuse by an adult child. Of those families, 197 reported a retraction of the abuse allegations by the accuser. Ten fathers from those 197 families were randomly selected and contacted for participation in a telephone interview. Of those 10, 1 declined and 2 could not be reached. Seven interviews were completed.

The hour-long interviews were conducted by the senior author

---

[1] The False Memory Syndrome Foundation is a nonprofit institution located at 3401 Market Street, Suite 130, Philadelphia, PA 19104. It was founded in March 1992 to study the origins of false memory syndrome and to disseminate scientific information on memory to the public and the professional community. The Foundation documents cases in which adults recover allegedly repressed memories and accuse their parents or others of sexually abusing them as children. The Foundation's Professional Advisory Board includes prominent researchers and clinicians from the fields of psychiatry, psychology, social work, law, and education.

(Harold Lief) and included questions that addressed the following areas: demographic information, details about the accusations and the retraction and the accused father's response to them, spouse and family reactions, and details about the effect on the accused (including emotional management, coping mechanisms, and impact on self-concept and on the social roles of husband and father).

Results

The respondents ranged in age from 58 to 72 years. All have had one marriage and remain married to the mother of the accusing child. Respondents came from a variety of professions: farming, military, and professional occupations. The range of allegations included vague impressions of sexual abuse or accusations of sexual abuse with no details given, to forced penetration from ages 2 to 16 years, to satanic ritual abuse, which included torture and violence. One respondent did not learn about the accusations against him until after his daughter realized that her memories of sexual abuse were false. All of the accusing daughters relinquished their memories as false.

Emotional Response to the Accusation

The most typical response to the accusations of sexual abuse was described as shock and disbelief. Respondents used words such as "numbness," "stunned," "shell shocked," and "frightened." Most fathers reported a complex reaction to the accusations. In some cases, this reaction was described as a progression of responses, as one father reported, from "hurt, to anger, to anguish, to wanting to know what happened, to frustration." Two fathers believed that clinical depression and, in one case, subsequent suicidal ideation were reactions to the accusations. One respondent had a stroke and one a heart attack after learning about the accusations—both reported feeling that their physical problems were exacerbated by the stress caused by the accusations.

Most of the respondents reported a type of "Job" reaction to the accusations (i.e., a search for an answer to the question, "Why me?"). In some cases this search led them to take action, which served as a coping mechanism. Others reported feeling over-whelmed by a sense of helplessness. An atypical response was one of being completely unflustered, almost detached, as one fa-ther reported.

Coping Mechanisms

All of the respondents made an attempt to understand what might have led their daughters to adopt the belief that their fa-ther had perpetrated sexual abuse. In some cases, this included a period of self-doubt, in which the father asked himself, "Could I have done this and be unaware of it?" In an attempt to answer this question, one father took a lie detector test. Another checked into a hospital to participate in treatment designed to access his own lost memories of having perpetrated sexual abuse. Others felt that a logical possibility for their daughters' memories of abuse might be that they were molested or otherwise sexually abused by someone else.

Several respondents reported seeking consultation with men-tal health professionals. One father felt that there was "a pre-sumption of guilt" by the psychiatrist with whom he met. Others found supportive mental health professionals.

Some respondents reported that they eventually experienced a sense of helplessness. One father said, "I couldn't do anything." Others took action in response to the accusations. This took the form of concentrating on work, reaching out for support (e.g., contacting the False Memory Syndrome Foundation), trying to learn about the issue, and even attempting to meet with the accus-ing daughter's therapist.

Respondents had to decide whether to disclose the accusa-tions to others or to conceal them. Even though most respon-dents reported an initial fear of disclosure, most decided to share their situation, often with close friends only. One father reported that he "told everyone." Although several respon-dents mentioned a connection to a church community as a source of support and as an aid in coping with the situation, one father was essentially shunned by his church and community after his daughter's therapist announced the accusations at an open church meeting.

Social Roles

Work.   In general, the accusations did not dramatically alter respondents' approach to work. (Two were retired at the time of the accusations.) Some respondents reported that they were less productive at work or completely unable to work for a period of time. One reported no change. Some reported the advantage of additional support from colleagues. In general, those who experienced some adverse effect on work life reported that it was short term.

Marriage.   Even though most respondents reported a fear that their spouse would be forced to choose between them and the accusing child, and that they would be rejected in this scenario, this fear was felt mostly in the initial period after the accusation and then subsided. Most respondents reported that ultimately they perceived their marriages as stronger because of this experience. They felt that the accusations served to draw them closer to their wives, in part to present a "united front" (this was especially true for those couples in which the wife was also accused of abuse or complicity). One father reported, "They were the best years of my marriage, in spite of the pain."

Some respondents reported that their marriage sustained a blow and that existing problems and differences were exacerbated. Even after the recantation, there were lingering doubts about the wife's loyalty. However, in all cases, respondents and their spouses remain married.

Parenting.   Respondents reported the need to search for what they had done wrong as parents and discussed the reevaluation of their fathering as part of the process of understanding how they could have been accused. In retrospect, some respondents felt that they could have been "better" fathers. "There are things I would do differently," one respondent said.

Some fathers reported that parental relationships were enhanced as a result of the accusation and retraction. In contrast, in several instances there was still a sense of alienation and distancing, possibly a result of underlying anger on the father's part and guilt on the daughter's part. In one case, in which the accusing daughter committed suicide after the retraction, the father developed a close relationship with her two sons, his grandchildren. In several cases the fathers felt much closer to their other children.

Self-concept.   Introspective data about a man's concept of himself are difficult to obtain in an abbreviated telephone interview. Nevertheless, we were left with strong impressions. A feeling of helplessness was almost universal, affecting the respondents' sense of power and strength. In some cases, especially if there was a prolonged period between the accusation and the recantation, this became a pervasive sense of self. This powerlessness is illustrated in one case in which the husband agreed to be separated from his wife for 7 months on the recommendation of a therapist. In most of the cases in which the retraction occurred within a year or two of the accusation, this diminished sense of strength was short-lived.

In this sample, the contrast between activity and passivity seemed significant. Some respondents succumbed to helplessness with passivity and even self-degradation as hallmarks of their behavior. Others, perhaps fueled by rage, struck back at the therapist whom they blamed for their misfortune. Several fathers reported that the sense of powerlessness was sometimes ameliorated by action. A few of the respondents became activists, fighting against the injustice, complaining to professional organizations, writing letters to elected officials, and writing letters to newspapers.

Some of the necessary affirmation of masculinity, such as a sense of being respected and powerful, was threatened by doubts about the wife's perception of the situation and by uncertainty about her belief in her husband's innocence. Only one father spontaneously mentioned that the accusations had an adverse effect on his sexual life. Half the respondents, however, were uncertain about their "head of household" role (these were traditional families) and felt that the accusations undermined their sense of power. With these men, even the retractions did not seem to correct the balance.

Limitations

This sample of men who faced an accusation of sexual abuse is clearly limited, and results cannot be generalized. The sample size is small and the group highly selected in that subjects were obtained from the False Memory Syndrome Foundation database. We can only discuss how these particular men responded to their situation. As with any retrospective self-report, there is always a question about the accuracy of the report. We did not rely on any objective measures of the elements we examined. Further, we also attempted to elicit introspective information from the respondents, and the men varied in their ability to provide this type of information. There are likely many factors influencing these men's interpretation of the events and their emotions surrounding the accusation and retraction.

Discussion

In this chapter, we have compared RMT with the formative years of psychoanalysis, in which the "talking cure," or abreaction, became the cornerstone of treatment. We have also noted how this approach became a treatment in which suggestion plays a dominant and ultimately harmful role in the process. Freud himself was cognizant of the dangers of suggestion and invented the psychoanalytic method, not only to help discover an individual's fantasy life but to decrease the power of suggestion. However, even in psychoanalysis, suggestion, including the implicit expectations of the analyst, is in play, and the circularity of interpretations and patient responses reinforces suggestion. We can recognize, then, how much more powerful suggestion is in nonanalytic therapeutic methods. RMT is described by Lear (1998) as "an often quackish practice in which so-called therapists actively encourage their clients to 'remember' incidents of abuse from childhood. After some initial puzzlement as to what is being asked of them, clients have been only too willing to oblige: inventing the wildest stories of satanic rituals, cannibalism . . . " (p. 21).

Although a number of legal cases have resulted in financial reward to the patient for years of RMT, it is not necessary to impugn the motives of therapists. Most cases of RMT are the consequence of ignorance or blind belief on the part of therapists and of the eagerness of clients to find meaning in their lives. In sheer numbers, psychiatrists have played a minor role in this travesty of psychotherapy—8% in one survey (Freyd et al. 1993), but because of the prestige or position of importance that psychiatrists have in the mental health establishment, their influence has been substantial. Several prominent psychiatrists have been involved in cases of dissociative identity disorder, including those with alleged satanic ritual abuse, and have been sued as a consequence. There's absolutely no evidence for satanic ritual abuse, which is often purported to include ritual torture, forced pregnancy, and child cannibalism (Lanning 1989; Victor 1993).

We have also provided additional documentation of the disastrous effects of RMT on the family, paying special attention to the impact on fathers accused by their adult daughters. For our study, we selected cases in which the daughter retracted her accusation, so that there was no remaining suspicion that these fathers were perpetrators of incest. The effect of the accusations on these men's self-concept is difficult to ascertain in the type of study we carried out, but it is fair to say that reactions ranged from devastation—including clinical depression and stroke, with inner feelings of helplessness, impotency, and despair—to one report of being relatively unfazed and almost untouched. Of the various coping mechanisms elucidated, activity, fighting back, and the search for group support were the most effective. These findings are consistent with other reports (de Rivera 1994; M. Elson, unpublished manuscript, 1998). For most fathers, the accusation became a defining moment in their lives.

It has been argued in some quarters that an attack on RMT is an attack on psychotherapy in general. To the contrary, our hope is to support effective therapy as strongly as we can. By demonstrating that RMT is a dangerous form of treatment, adversely affecting the lives of the patients subjected to these techniques, and having a catastrophic effect on the family, we wish to enable professionals and their patients to discriminate between "good" and "bad" psychotherapy. Any "good" psychotherapy has to help patients to understand and, if they wish, change their irrational and maladaptive behavior patterns. This can be done without recourse to pseudo-memories of trauma. There is enough genuine trauma to go around.

Conclusion

As many professional organizations have stated, RMT should be avoided. The consequences to the primary patient have been reported in many contributions, including our own. A great deal of attention has been paid in the popular press to the consequences of false accusations, but less attention has been paid in the professional literature to the impact of false accusations on family members. Our preliminary study provides some understanding of the effects on false allegations of sexual abuse on the accused father.

It is clear that a significant event like this becomes a defining feature of a man's life. This can be injurious at any time. The men in our sample were at similar developmental stages. They were retired or close to retirement. Instead of experiencing peace and tranquility and enjoying their children and grandchildren, as they anticipated, they were hit with a bombshell that had disastrous consequences. Even where the accuser retracts the allegations, things are never quite the same. That sentiment was echoed with sadness by the men we interviewed.

References

Althaus v. Cohen, 1998 PA Super. Lexis 631—(Appellate) Ct. of Common Pleas, Allegheny Co., Penn., No. GD. 92–20893

American Medical Association: Memories of childhood sexual abuse: report of the Council on Scientific Affairs. CSA 5-A-94, 1994

American Psychiatric Association: Statement on memories of sexual abuse. December 1993

American Psychological Association: Questions and answers about memories of childhood abuse. August 1995

Australian Psychological Society Limited: Guidelines relating to the reporting of recovered memories. October 1994

Bass E, Davis L: The Courage to Heal: A Guide for Women Survivors of Child Sexual Abuse. New York, Harper & Row, 1988

Brandon S, Boakes J, Glaser D, et al: Reported recovered memories of child sexual abuse: recommendations for good practice and implications for training, continuing professional development and research. Psychiatr Bull 21:663–665, 1997

Brenneis CB: Recovered Memories of Trauma: Transferring the Present to the Past. Madison, WI, International Universities Press, 1997

Canadian Psychiatric Association: Position statement: adult recovered memories of childhood sexual abuse. Can J Psychiatry 41:305–306, 1996

De Rivera J: Impact of child abuse memories on the families of victims. Issues in Child Abuse Accusations 6:149–155, 1994

De Rivera J: The construction of false memory syndrome: the experience of retractors. Psychological Inquiry 8:271–291, 1997

DuChateau C: Recovered memory or just a giant con trick? New Zealand Herald, September 9, 1998, p A13

False Memory Syndrome Foundation: Family survey update. FMSF Newsletter, April 1997

Fetkewicz JM, Sharma V, Merskey H: A note on suicidal deterioration with recovered memory treatment. J Affect Disord (in press)

Frederickson R: Repressed Memories: A Journey to Recovery From Sexual Abuse. New York, Simon & Schuster, 1992

Freud S: An Autobiographical Study. London, Hogarth Press, 1946

Freud S: Constructions in analysis (1938), in The Standard Edition of the Complete Psychological Works of Sigmund Freud, Vol 23. Translated and edited by Strachey J. London, Hogarth Press, 1964, pp 255–296

Freyd P, Roth A, Wakefield H, et al: Results of the False Memory Syndrome Foundation family survey. Paper presented at Memory and Reality: Emerging Crisis Conference, Valley Forge, PA, April 1993

Fultz v. Carr and Walker, Circuit Ct., Multnomah Co., Oregon. No. 9506–04080

Garry M, Manning CG, Loftus EF, et al: Imagination inflation: imagining a childhood event inflates confidence that it occurred. Psychonomic Bulletin 3:208–214, 1996

Gavigan M: False memories of childhood sexual abuse: a personal account. Issues in Child Abuse Accusations 4:246–247, 1992

Goldberg L: A psychoanalytic look at recovered memories, therapists, cult leaders, and undue influence. Clinical Social Work Journal 25:71–86, 1997

Goldstein E, Farmer K: Confabulations. Boca Raton, FL, Sirs Publishing, 1992

Goldstein E, Farmer K: True Stories of False Memories. Boca Raton, FL, Sirs Publishing, 1993

Goodyear-Smith FA, Laidlaw TM, Large RG: Surveying families accused of childhood sexual abuse: a comparison of British and New Zealand results. Applied Cognitive Psychology 11:31–34, 1997

Gudjonsson GH: The members of the British false memory society, the accusers and their siblings. The Psychologist 10(3):111–115, 1997

Herman JL, Schatzow E: Recovery and verification of memories of childhood sexual trauma. Psychoanal Psychol 4:1–14, 1987

Holmes DS: The evidence for repression: an examination of sixty years of research, in Repression and Dissociation. Edited by Singer JL. Chicago, IL, University of Chicago Press, 1990, pp 85–102

Hughes R: Culture of Complaint: The Fraying of America. New York, Oxford University Press, 1993

Karlin RA, Orne MT: Commentary on *Borawick v. Shay:* hypnosis, social influence, incestuous child abuse and satanic ritual abuse; the iatrogenic creation of horrific memories for the remote past. Cultic Studies Journal 13:42–93, 1996

Kihlstrom JF: Exhumed memory, in Truth in Memory. Edited by Lynn SJ, McConkey KM. New York, Guilford, 1998, pp 3–31

Lanning KS: Satanic, occult, ritualistic crime: a law enforcement perspective. The Police Chief, October 1989, p 62

Lear J: Open Minded. Cambridge, MA, Harvard University Press, 1998

Lief HI, Fetkewicz JM: Retractors of false memories: the evolution of pseudomemories. Journal of Psychiatry and Law 23:411–435, 1995

Lindsay DS, Read JD: Psychotherapy and memories of childhood sexual abuse. Applied Cognitive Psychology 8:281–338, 1994

Lindsay DS, Read JD: "Memory work" and recovered memories of childhood sexual abuse: scientific evidence and public, professional and personal issues. Psychology, Public Policy, and the Law 1: 846–908, 1995

Loftus EF: The reality of repressed memories. Am Psychol 48:518–535, 1993

Loftus EF, Ketchum K: The Myth of Repressed Memories: False Memories and Allegations of Sexual Abuse. New York, St. Martin's, 1994

Marietti et al. v. Kluft et al., Ct. of Common Pleas, Phila Co. Penn. No. 9509–02260

Marmor J: Limitations of free association. Arch Gen Psychiatry 22: 160–164, 1970

Masson J: The Assault on the Truth. New York, Farrar Strauss Giroux, 1984

McElroy SL, Keck PE: The formation of false memories. Psychiatr Ann 25:720–725, 1995

Nelson EL, Simpson P: First glimpse: an initial examination of subjects who have rejected their visualizations as false memories. Issues in Child Abuse Accusations 6:123–133, 1994

Ofshe R, Watters E: Making Monsters: False Memory, Psychotherapy and Sexual Hysteria. New York, Scribner, 1994

Pasley L: Misplaced trust: a first person account of how my therapist created false memories. Skeptic 2:62–67, 1994

Pendergrast M: Victims of Memory: Incest Accusations and Shattered Lives, 2nd Ed. Hinesburg, VT, Upper Access Books, 1996

Perry C: The false memory syndrome (FMS) and "disguised" hypnosis. Hypnos 22:189–198, 1995

Piper A: What science says—and doesn't say—about repressed memories: a critique of Scheflin and Brown. Journal of Psychiatry and Law 24:615–639, 1996

Poole DA, Lindsay DS, Memon A, et al: Psychotherapy and the recovery of memories of childhood sexual abuse: U.S. and British practitioners' beliefs, practices and experiences. J Consult Clin Psychol 63:426–437, 1995

Pope HG, Hudson JL: Can memories of childhood sexual abuse be repressed? Psychol Med 25:121–126, 1995

Pope HG, Hudson JI, Bodkin JA, et al: Questionable validity of 'dissociative amnesia' in trauma victims: evidence from prospective studies. Br J Psychiatry 172:210–215, 1998

Scheflin AW, Brown D: Repressed memory or dissociate amnesia: what the science says. Journal of Psychiatry and Law 24:143–188, 1996

Shorter E: From Paralysis to Fatigue: A History of Psychosomatic Illness in the Modern Era. New York, Free Press, 1992

Sifford D: Accusations of sex abuse, years later. Philadelphia Inquirer, November 24, 1991, p F1

Sommers CH: Who Stole Feminism: How Women Have Betrayed Women. New York, Simon & Schuster, 1994

Steinfels P: Cardinal Bernardin dies at 68; reconciling voice in church. The New York Times, November 15, 1996, pp A1/A17

United States of America v. Peterson et al., US District Court, Southern Dist., Texas, No. H-97–237

Victor JS: Satanic Panic. Chicago, IL, Open Court, 1993

Woodward KL, McCormick J: The art of dying well. Newsweek, November 25, 1996, pp 61–67

Wright L: Remembering Satan: Case of Recovered Memory and the Shattering of an American Family. New York, Knopf, 1994

Yapko M: Suggestions of Abuse: True and False Memories of Childhood Sexual Trauma. New York, Simon & Schuster, 1994

Afterword

Richard C. Friedman, M.D., and
Jennifer I. Downey, M.D.

The chapters in this volume discuss different dimensions of masculinity and male sexuality. A perspective they share is that biological, psychological, and social influences on behavior must be conceptualized from a developmental perspective in order to adequately assess sexual function and treat difficulties and disorders. The topics reviewed are not restricted in their relevance to patients of a particular diagnosis or group of diagnoses, but rather they shed light on clinical issues important to all male patients.

The chapters by Friedman and Downey, Levine, and Althof and Seftel may be construed as a larger unit, each discussing different aspects of male erotic experience. The most important subtext of the chapter by Friedman and Downey is that it is not possible to adequately understand a male psychotherapy patient without assessing the meaning of his sexual experience and activity. Levine broadens the canvas by including the subject of love, not merely sex. The psychology of sexual love has long resisted the efforts of clinicians to understand it and of scientists to illuminate its origins. Steadfastly refusing to be intimidated by the complexity of his topic, Levine argues that impediments in the development of the capacity to sexually love lead to diverse psychiatric difficulties. Whether symptom relief (e.g., in depression or anxiety) can be effected and sustained without adequate repair of underlying deficits in the capacity to love remains to be determined by research. In any case, relatively few modern clinicians probably know whether their male patients love anyone or have ever fallen in love, nor do they know their male patients' ideas about sexual love. A clinical database about love remains to be established.

Althof and Seftel's chapter makes different demands on the reader. In order to understand sexual function and dysfunction, it is necessary to be knowledgeable about not only psychology but also physiology. Their chapter, which begins with nosology, epidemiology, and physiology, concludes with a discussion of the psychology of people—individuals and couples. Substantial knowledge and skill are required to treat sexual difficulties in men and women, and cross-disciplinary approaches have often proven helpful.

The last two chapters direct the reader's attention toward different aspects of fatherhood, a topic underemphasized by Freud and traditional psychoanalytic theoreticians. Pollack presents a psychodynamically informed discussion of phase-specific, life cycle issues. He emphasizes the positive aspects of fatherhood and provides a model for conceptualizing "good-enough fathering." Lief and Fetkewicz focus on a painful and distressing derailment of normal family life: fathers who have been falsely accused of having sexually abused their daughters. This group has not been discussed extensively in the psychiatric literature, and Lief and Fetkewicz's chapter is the beginning of a more extensive investigation of an important subject.

This special volume illustrates the usefulness and importance of examining clinical issues pertaining to human sexuality from a biopsychosocial perspective, in addition to using the more limited medical model that informs the *Diagnostic and Statistical Manual of Mental Disorders,* Fourth Edition (Engel 1977). Male sexuality is only one of many areas whose study indicates that, in order to effectively relieve symptoms, it is necessary to understand and provide treatment to the patients in whom these symptoms occur.

Reference

Engel G: The need for a new medical model: a challenge for biomedicine. Science 196:129, 1977

Index

*Page numbers printed in **boldface** type refer to tables or figures.*

Adolescents and adolescence. *See also* Children and childhood
heterosexual development and, 30–31, 33–34
sexual desire and sexual activity in, 13
Adrenarche, 30
Adults, and heterosexual development, 31
Advanced glycation end-products (AGEs), 62, 63
Affiliation, and concept of self, 97–98, 111–113
Age and aging, and erectile dysfunction, 58, 62–63
Aggression
destructive sexual activity and, 16
heterosexual development and, 43–44
rejection and, 34–35
Alienation, in sexual relationships, 45
Allergies, and erectile dysfunction, 58
Althaus v. Cohen, 131
American Psychiatric Association, on recovered memory therapy, 119
Amnesia, 118
Amyl nitrate, 70
Anatomy, and physiology of erection, 58–59

Androgens. *See also* Testosterone
adolescence and sexual development, 30
erectile dysfunction and index of stimulation, 68
sexual drive and, 38
Anemia, and hypoxemia, 63–64
Anhedonia, 41
Anticonvulsants, 39
Antihypertensive agents
erectile dysfunction and, 58
sexual drive and, 39
Antipsychotic medications, and erectile dysfunction, 58
Antisocial behavior, and destructive sexual activity, 16
Antisocial personality disorder, 21
Anxiety
sexual arousal and, 15
sexual fantasies and countertransference, 12–13
Aphrodisiacs, 39
Apomorphine (TAP), 71
Arthritis, and erectile dysfunction, 58
Atypical bipolar disorder, and hypersexuality, 14
Autonomy, and concept of self, 97–98, 111–113

Behavior
adolescence and sexual development, 30–31

Behavior *(continued)*
  destructive sexual activity and
    antisocial, 16
  proto-heterosexuality in male
    children and, 30
Biology, and sexual drive, 38–39
Biopsychosocial perspective, on
  sexuality, 144
Bipolar II disorder, and
  hypersexuality, 14
Bisexuality. *See also* Sexual
  orientation
  identity issues and personality
    disorders, 22–23
  sexual fantasies and, 5
Borderline personality disorder,
  22–23
Boston University Pregnancy and
  Parenthood Project (BUPP),
  91, 96–97, 102, 104–107
Boundary violations, and sexual
  impulsivity or compulsivity,
  19
BUPP (Boston University
  Pregnancy and Parenthood
  Project), 91, 96–97, 102,
  104–107
Bupropion, 39

Cardiac drugs, and erectile
  dysfunction, 58
Cavernosal arteries, 59, 61
Celibacy, and sexual fantasies, 6
Children and childhood. *See also*
  Adolescents and adolescence;
  Development; Recovered
  memory therapy; Sexual
  abuse
  function of fantasy in, 1
  gender and identity formation
    in, 92–96

proto-heterosexuality and
  behavior of, 30
Cholesterol, levels of and erectile
  dysfunction, 58
Cigarette smoking, and erectile
  dysfunction, 58
Cimetidine, 39
Clinical issues, in male sexuality.
  See also Psychotherapy
  biopsychosocial perspective
    and, 144
  personality disorders and,
    21–23
  sexual fantasy and, 1–6, 13
  sexual impulsivity or
    compulsivity and, 14–21
  sexuality in psychotherapeutic
    context and, 6–13
  sexual orientation conversion
    and, 23–24
Collagen, aging and erectile
  dysfunction, 62
Combined treatment, and
  psychotherapy, 7
Communication skills, and
  psychological intimacy, 48
Complementarity, in parenting,
  99
Compulsions, and destructive
  sexual activities, 15. *See also*
  Sexual impulsivity and
  compulsivity
Conversation, and psychological
  intimacy, 48–49
Coping skills and styles
  false accusations of childhood
    sexual abuse and, 130,
    133, 137
  sexual arousal and, 15
Core gender identity, 110–111
Corpora cavernosa, 58–59

Corporal veno-occlusive
mechanism, 61
Corpus spongiosum, 58–59
Countertransference, and sexual
fantasies, 9–13
Couples therapy
erectile dysfunction and, 73, 80
sex differences and, 4–5
Crime, and sexual aggression, 44.
See also Violence
Culture
physical appearance of women
and, 46
sexual expectations and, 41
Cyproterone acetate, 2

Default heterosexuality, 32–36
Depression, and sexual motives,
41
Destructive sexual activity, as
clinical issue, 14–16
Detumescence, and physiology of
erection, 61
Development. *See also* Children
and childhood
autonomy and concept of the
self, 96–98
common manifestations of
heterosexual failure,
42–46
concept of heterosexual
failure, 36–42
fathering as phase of, 101–104
gender and identity formation,
92–96
normal process of
heterosexual, 30–32
Diabetes, and erectile
dysfunction, 58, 62–63
Diagnosis
of erectile dysfunction, 66–68

of male erectile disorder, **57**
sexual motivations and, 16
*Diagnostic and Statistical Manual of
Mental Disorders,* Fourth
Edition (American
Psychiatric Association, 1994)
dissociative amnesia and,
118
levels of impairment in
patients seeking
psychotherapy, 7
male erectile disorder and,
56–57
medical model of sexuality
and, 144
Digitalis, 39
Dissociative amnesia, 118
Dissociative identity disorder,
127, 137
Don Juanism, 44
Dosage, of sildenafil citrate, 71
Dreams, recovered memory
therapy and interpretation of,
125–126
Drop-out rates, from therapy for
erectile dysfunction, 79,
80–81
DSM-IV. *See Diagnostic and
Statistical Manual of Mental
Disorders,* Fourth Edition
Duplicity, patterns of in sexual
behavior, 44–45

Education, and treatment of
erectile dysfunction, 69, 73
Emotions, and fathers falsely
accused of sexual abuse, 130,
132–133
Endothelin, 59–60, 64
Erectile dysfunction
future of therapy for, 81

Erectile dysfunction (continued)
   interactive etiologic model
      paradigm for, 65–66
   mental health clinicians and,
      78–81
   nosology of impotence and,
      56–57
   physiology of erection, 58–65
   prevalence of and medical risk
      factors for, 57–65
   process of care model for,
      66–78
   sildenafil citrate and, 55,
      70–71, 81
   treatment of, 55–56, 65–81
   wish component of sexual
      drive and, 42
Eroticization, and psychological
   intimacy, 49–50
Estrogens, 39
Extramarital affairs. See also
   Marriage
   heterosexual development and
      patterns of repeated,
      45
   sexual impulsivity or
      compulsivity and,
      19

False memory syndrome,
   120–122
False Memory Syndrome
   Foundation, 131, 136
Family. See also Parents and
   parenting
   false allegations of childhood
      sexual abuse and, 117,
      128–131
   structure of and styles of
      parenting, 99
Fantasy. See Sexual fantasy

Fathers and fatherhood. See also
   Parents and parenting;
   Recovered memories; Sexual
   abuse
   autonomy-affiliation balance
      and concept of self, 98,
      111–113
   concept of as transformation of
      self, 89–92
   development and, 101–104
   family structure and styles of,
      99–101
   impact of false accusations of
      sexual abuse on, 128–131
   inhibitions and interruptions
      in transition to, 107–109
   interviews with fathers falsely
      accused of sexual abuse,
      131–136
   needs of men and boys,
      109–111
   personal experiences of,
      104–107
   recommendations on, 111–113
Feminist theory
   on gender and development,
      92, 110
   recovered memory therapy
      and, 126–127
Fetishism, 36
Fluoxetine, 39
Fluvoxamine, 39
Follow-up studies, of
      psychotherapy for erectile
      dysfunction, 74–75
Freud, Sigmund, 1–2, 6, 9, 20,
      24–25, 93, 122–123, 126, 136
Fultz v. Carr and Walker, 131

GAF (Global Assessment of
   Functioning) Scale, 7

Gap junctions, and physiology of erection, 62
Gender. *See also* Sex differences; Women
  autonomy-affiliation balance and styles of parenting, 98
  identity formation and, 92–96, 110–111
  influence of roles and expectations on parenting, 99
Generativity, and fathering, 102
Gene therapy, and erectile dysfunction, 64–65
Global Assessment of Functioning (GAF) Scale, 7
Gonadarche, 30
Good-enough fathering, 101–104
Guilt, and sexual fantasies and activity, 16–18

Health care system, and psychotherapy, 8, 25
Heart disease, and erectile dysfunction, 58
Heterosexuality, male. *See also* Sexual orientation
  basic concepts in, 29
  common manifestations of developmental failures, 42–46
  concept of failure, 36–42
  default form of, 32–36
  intimacy skills and, 47–52
  normal process of development, 30–32
  sexual fantasies and, 5–6, 13
  sexual orientation conversion and, 23–24

Homophobia
  countertransference issues in psychotherapy and, 11
  sexual impulsivity or compulsivity and internalized, 20–21
  sexual orientation conversion and internalized, 24
Homosexuality, male. *See also* Sexual orientation
  countertransference issues in psychotherapy and, 10–11, 11–12, 13
  internalized homophobia and, 20–21, 24
  sexual fantasies and, 5–6, 13
  sexual orientation conversion and, 23–24
Hostility, and sexual arousal, 15
Hypersexuality, 14
Hypertension, and erectile dysfunction, 58
Hypoglycemic agents, and erectile dysfunction, 58
Hypomania, and hypersexuality, 14
Hypoxemia, and erectile dysfunction, 63–64

Identity
  bisexuality and, 22–23
  gender and formation of, 92–96, 110–111
Impotence, 56–57. *See also* Erectile dysfunction
Incest. *See* Sexual abuse
Inflatable penile prosthesis, 78
Infrastructure, of heterosexuality, 35–36
Inhibition, and internalized homophobia, 21

Initial assessment, and sexual history, 7–9

Interactive paradigm, of erectile dysfunction, 65–66

Internalization, and psychological intimacy, 49

Intimacy, heterosexuality and skills of psychological, 47–52

Intracavernosal self-injection therapy, 75–76

Laboratory tests, and erectile dysfunction, 69

Lacunar spaces, of penis, 59, 60–61

Language, and intimacy skills, 47–48

Learning, and relationship between sexual desire and activity, 13

Legal cases, and recovered memories of childhood sexual abuse, 130–131, 136–137

Life cycle
fatherhood and, 107–109
male heterosexual, 32
sexual fantasies and, 3–4

Loss, of psychological intimacy, 50–51

Male erectile disorder, 56–57

Malleable penile prosthesis, 78

Mania, and hypersexuality, 14

Marietti et al. v. Kluft et al., 131

Marriage. *See also* Extramarital affairs; Relationships
countertransference issues in psychotherapy and, 11–12

false accusations of sexual abuse and, 134

Masculinity. *See* Gender; Heterosexuality; Sexuality

Massachusetts Male Aging Study, 57–58

Medical conditions
erectile dysfunction and, 58, 70–72
sexual motives and illness in partner, 40

Medicated urethral system for erection (MUSE), 76–77

Medications. *See also* Psychopharmacology
erectile dysfunction and, 58, 68
sexual drive and, 39

Mental health
fatherhood and, 103
sexual fantasies and, 24–25

Methylphenidate, 39

Mixed erectile disorder, 65

Mood disorders, and destructive sexual activities, 15

Morality, and countertransference issues in psychotherapy, 10–11

Moral masochism, 20

Mothers and motherhood, and role of gender in identity formation, 94–96. *See also* Parents and parenting

Multiple personality disorder. *See* Dissociative identity disorder

MUSE (medicated urethral system for erection), 76–77

Narcissism, and heterosexual development, 45

Narcissistic personality disorder, 21, 96

National Institutes of Health, 56
Neuroendocrinology, and sexual
    drive, 38–39
Neurologic examination, and
    erectile dysfunction, 68
Neurovascular factors, and
    physiology of erection, 59–61
Nitric oxide, and physiology of
    erection, 60, 61–62
Nitric oxide synthase (NOS)
    enzymes, 61–62
Nonadrenergic-noncholinergic
    (NANC) nerves, 60
Nosology, of impotence and
    erectile dysfunction, 56–57

Oedipus complex, 93
Opioids, 39

Papaverine hydrochloride,
    75
Paraphilias
    sexual drive and, 41
    sexual fantasies and, 3
    sexual masochism and, 20
    treatment of, 16
Parents and parenting. See also
    Family; Fathers and
    fatherhood; Mothers and
    motherhood
    adolescents and sexual
        development, 31
    false accusations of sexual
        abuse and, 134–135
Paroxetine, 39
Pathophysiology, of erectile
    dysfunction, 62–63
Penile prosthesis, 77–78
Penis, and physiology of erection,
    58–59
Pentosidine, 63

Performance anxiety, and erectile
    dysfunction, 67
Personality disorders
    clinical issues in severe cases
        of, 21–23
    destructive sexual activity and,
        15
Peyronie's disease, 68
Phenothiazines, 39
Phentolamine, 75
Physical examination, and
    erectile dysfunction, 68–69
Physiology, of erection, 58–65
Power, heterosexuality and
    inequities of, 35–36
Prevalence
    of dissociative identity
        disorder, 127
    of erectile dysfunction, 57–58
Process of care (POC) model, for
    erectile dysfunction, 66–78
Progesterone, 39
Prostaglandin, 75, 76
Proto-heterosexuality, 30
Pseudo-memories, and recovered
    memory therapy, 120–122,
    124
Psyche, and psychological
    intimacy, 49
Psychopharmacology, and
    combined treatment, 7.
    See also Medications
Psychotherapy. See also Clinical
    issues
    erectile dysfunction and, 56,
        65, 72–75
    health care system and, 8, 25
    recovered memory therapy
        and, 136–138
    sexual issues in context of,
        6–13

Pulmonary hypoxemia, 63

Recovered memory therapy
(RMT), and false accusations
of childhood sexual abuse.
See also Sexual abuse
dissociative amnesia and, 118
mutually reinforcing beliefs
and, 124–126
psychotherapy and, 136–138
retractors of false memories
and, 120–122
role of suggestion in, 123–124,
125, 136
theoretical issues in, 122–123
therapeutic assumptions of,
118–120, 126–127
Rectal examination, and erectile
dysfunction, 69
Rejection, and aggression, 34–35
Relationships. *See also* Marriage;
Social interaction
adults and sexual
development, 31
erectile dysfunction and,
67–68
heterosexual development
and, 44, 45
psychological intimacy and,
50, 51
sexual impulsivity or
compulsivity and
undermining of, 19–20
Renal failure, and hypoxemia,
64
Repression, of memories of
sexual abuse, 117–118
Retractors, of false memories of
sexual abuse, 120–122
Royal College of Psychiatrists,
119

Sadomasochism, and power
inequity, 35–36
Secondary sex characteristics, 68
Selective serotonin reuptake
inhibitors (SSRIs)
erectile dysfunction and, 58
sexual drive and, 39
Self
false accusations of sexual
abuse and concept of,
135, 137
gender and development of,
96–98, 111–113
Self-esteem
fatherhood and, 105–106
sexuality and sex differences
in, 5
Self-help movement, and
recovered memory therapy,
126
Self-injection, as therapy for
erectile dysfunction, 75–76
Sertraline, 39
Sex differences, and sexual
fantasies, 4–5. *See also* Gender
Sexual abuse, false accusations of
childhood and recovered
memories. *See also* Recovered
memory therapy
false memory syndrome and,
120–122
family relationships and, 117,
128–131
impact of accusations on
fathers, 128–131
interviews with accused
fathers, 131–136
public and media attention to
cases of, 115
repressed memories and,
117–120

victims with continuous memories and, 116
Sexual addicts, 15–16
Sexual arousal, and sexual desire, 37
Sexual counseling, for erectile dysfunction, 72–75
Sexual desire
  biological component of, 38–39
  oversimplification of concept, 37–38
  psychological component of, 39–41
  social component of, 41–42
Sexual drive, as biological component of sexual desire, 38–39
  psychological component of, 39–41
Sexual dysfunction
  due to a general medical condition, 57
  in partner and erectile dysfunction, 67–68
Sexual fantasy
  default heterosexuality and, 35
  destructive sexual activity and, 14, 15
  forms of, 2–4
  general aspects of, 1–2
  mental health and, 24–25
  moral masochism and, 20
  psychotherapy and countertransference, 9–13
  sexual activity and, 13
  sex differences in, 4–5
  sexual orientation and, 5–6, 23–24
Sexual function, and psychological intimacy, 51–52

Sexual guilt, and sexual impulsivity or compulsivity, 16
Sexual history, and psychotherapy, 7–9
Sexual impulsivity and compulsivity. See also Compulsions
  boundary violations and, 19
  destructive sexual activity and, 14–16
  Freud's concepts of moral masochism and sexual masochism and, 20
  internalized homophobia and, 20–21
  sexual guilt and, 16–18
  undermining of relationships and, 19–20
Sexuality, male. See also Clinical issues; Erectile dysfunction; Fathers and fatherhood; Heterosexuality
  biopsychosocial perspective versus medical model of, 144
  importance of to mental health, 24–25
Sexual masochism, 20
Sexual motivations
  diagnosis of psychopathology and, 16
  psychological component of sexual desire and, 39–41
Sexual orientation. See also Bisexuality; Heterosexuality; Homosexuality
  conversion and, 23–24
  sexual fantasies and, 5–6
Sexual response, dual-control system of, 81

Sexual wish, 41–42
Shame, and sexual fantasies, 2
Side effects, of treatments for
    erectile dysfunction
    sildenafil citrate, 70, **71**
    self-injection therapy, 76, **77**
    transurethral therapy, 77, **78**
    vacuum tumescence therapy,
        72
Sildenafil citrate (Viagra), 55,
    70–71, 81
Social interaction. *See also*
    Relationships
    fathers and false accusations of
        sexual abuse, 134–135
    sexual drive and skills in,
        40
    sexual relationships and
        deficits in, 44
    sexual wish and, 41–42
Spironolactone, 39
Splitting, sexual fantasies and
    countertransference, 11
SSRIs. *See* Selective serotonin
    reuptake inhibitors
Subgroups, and types of sexual
    fantasies, 3
Substance abuse
    destructive sexual activities
        and, 15
    sexual drive and, 39
Substance-induced sexual
    dysfunction, 57
Suggestion, and recovered
    memory therapy, 123–124,
    125, 136
Symptoms, sexual fantasies and
    intractable nonsexual, 11

Testosterone, 39, 40. *See also*
    Androgens

Therapist. *See*
    Countertransference;
    Psychotherapy; Transference
Trauma
    gender and developmental,
        94–96
    recovered memory therapy
        and, 122
Transference
    Freud and definition of, 6
    psychological intimacy and,
        49
Transurethral therapy, for erectile
    dysfunction, 76–77
Transvestic fetishism, 36
Trazodone, 39
Tricyclic antidepressants, and
    erectile dysfunction, 58
Trimix, and injection therapy for
    erectile dysfunction, 75
Tunica albuginea, 59

Ulcers, and erectile dysfunction,
    58
Urologic history, and erectile
    dysfunction, 68–69

Vacuum tumescence therapy, 72
Values and value system
    internalized homophobia and,
        20–21
    sexual fantasies and
        countertransference,
        11–12
    sexual orientation conversion
        and, 24
Vascular examination, and
    erectile dysfunction, 68–69
Vasodilators, and erectile
    dysfunction, 58
Vasomax, 71

Viagra (sildenafil citrate), 55, 70–71, 81
Violence, and destructive sexual activities or fantasies, 16. *See also* Crime

Women. *See also* Gender
    autonomy-affiliation balance and concept of self, 98
    psychological intimacy and, 51

sexual development in males and attitudes toward, 31–32
sexual drives and motives of, 40
sexual fantasy and, 4–5
Work, and fathers
    false accusations of sexual abuse and, 134
    parenting roles and, 100, 106

Yohimbine, 39, 71–72